Copyright 2020 by Thomas Anderson -All rights reserved.

No part of this book may be reproduced or transmitted in any form or by any means, electronic or mechanical, including photocopying and recording, or by any information storage and retrieval system, without permission in writing from the publisher. This is a work of fiction. Names, places, characters and incidents are either the product of the author's imagination or are used fictitiously, and any resemblance to any actual persons, living or dead, organizations, events or locales is entirely coincidental. The unauthorized reproduction or distribution of this copyrighted work is ilegal.

Disclaimer Notice:

Please note the information contained within this document is for educational and entertainment purposes only. All effort has been executed to present accurate, up to date, reliable, complete information. No warranties of any kind are declared or implied. Readers acknowledge that the author is not engaged in the rendering of legal, financial, medical, or professional advice. The content within this book has been derived from various sources. Please consult a licensed professional before attempting any techniques outlined in this book.

By reading this document, the reader agrees that under no circumstances is the author responsible for any losses, direct or indirect, that are incurred as a result of the use of the information contained within this document, including, but not limited to, errors, omissions, or inaccuracies.

CONTENTS

- INTRODUCTION 4
  - WHAT IS JACKFRUIT 4
  - HEALTH BENEFITS OF JACKFRUIT 5
  - SUSTAINABLE FOOD SOURCE 6
  - HOW TO PREPARE 6
  - WHERE TO BUY 6
- RECIPES 7
  - CHICK'N & SWEET CORN SOUP 7
  - HOT & SOUR WONTON SOUP 8
  - CHICK'N NOODLE SOUP 9
  - GOULASH SOUP 10
  - TOONA MELT SANDWICH 11
  - PHILLY CHEEZESTEAK 12
  - THE VEGAN CUBAN 13
  - SLOW-COOKER REUBEN 14
  - CRISPY CHICK'N NUGGETS 15
  - BBQ PULLED-NOT-PORK BURGER 16
  - SMOKY CHICK'N SALAD 17
  - TOONA COLLARD WRAPS 18
  - VEGAN QUICHE LORRAINE 19
  - VIETNAMESE SALAD 20
  - NICOISE SALAD 21
  - SLOW-COOKER CHILLI 22
  - BBQ PULLED-NOT-PORK TACOS 23
  - MAC 'N' CHEEZE 24
  - TOONA PASTA BAKE 25
  - HAWAIIAN PIZZA 26
  - SUSHI ROLLS 27
  - VIETNAMESE ROLLS WITH PEANUT DIP 28
  - SWEET AND STICKY CHINESE JACKFRUIT 29
  - CRISPY PEKING JACK PANCAKES 30
  - STEAMED CHAR SIU BAO BUNS 31
  - SWEET AND SOUR JACKFRUIT 32
  - BUTTER CHICK'N 33
  - VEGAN MADRAS 34
  - SRI-LANKAN COCONUT CURRY 35
  - BANGLADESHI BIRYANI 36
  - NANKA RENDANG 37

INTRODUCTION

I am infatuated with jackfruit. The more I make with it, the more ideas I come up with for dishes to use it in. I first discovered it 7 years ago whilst travelling in Asia and was fascinated by its deliciousness and convincing meat-like texture; I genuinely believed I was eating pulled pork! Since then, it has become a hit with the vegan community as a meat-substitute and is popping up on supermarket shelves and restaurant menus all over the UK.

Jackfruit is a healthy and completely sustainable meat replacement. There are many other meat substitutes available nowadays, ranging from gluten-based seitan, to soy-based tofu, to the wide variety of Quorn products on offer. But jackfruit wins hands down. It is all natural, non-processed and its fibrous flesh can take on almost any flavour.

Here are just some of the reasons to love jackfruit:
- No cholesterol
- No saturated fat
- High in fibre
- High in potassium
- Low calorie
- Affordable
- Sustainable
- Ethical
- Versatile

This book contains over 50 vegan recipes to inspire you to use this magical fruit. From soups to sandwiches, stews to spring rolls, you will see how delicious and versatile jackfruit can be. All recipes use canned young, green jackfruit – the savoury kind that is most commonly found outside of tropical climates.

WHAT IS JACKFRUIT

Jackfruit is an enormous, green and knobbly fruit with a pale-yellow flesh inside. It's the biggest fruit in the world and can weigh up to 100lbs (45kg)! It's a tropical fruit that is related to figs, mulberry, and breadfruit. The jackfruit plant originated in southwest India, but is also grown across other tropical climates in Southeast Asia, the East Indies, Africa, South America, and Hawaii.

Depending on the ripeness of the fruit, you will get different flavours and textures. Young, green jackfruit (what we use in this book) has a mild flavour that melds well with a variety of seasonings. It is also stringy (in a good way) so it shreds easily to resemble the texture of meat. When the jackfruit is ripe, it has a sweet taste (and peculiar smell) and can be used in desserts and smoothies.

It is the national fruit of Bangladesh and has long been used in Asian cooking before it gained traction as a vegan meat substitute.

GREEN THAI CURRY	38
JAMAICAN JERK JACKFRUIT	39
JERK BLACK BEAN AND MANGO WRAP	40
NOT-JUST-MUSHROOM STROGANOFF	41
VEGAN GYROS	42
JACKFRUIT 'LAMB' TAGINE	43
NANA'S HOT POT	44
CHICK'N AND MUSHROOM PIE	45
GUINESSS IRISH STEW	46
JACKFRUIT AND STOUT COTTAGE PIE	47
STUFFED PEPPERS	48
LOADED NACHOS	49
JACK AND THE BLACK BEANS ENCHILADAS	50
SLOW-COOKER STUFFED SWEET POTATOES	51
SWEET CHILLI SPRING ROLLS	52
SMOKY PULLED-NOT-PORK TACOS	53
MEATLESS TIKKA MASALA	54
STICKY JACKFRUIT RIBS	55
TERIYAKI BOWL	56
FISH-FREE FINGERS AND CHIPS	57
THAI FISH-FREE CAKES	58

HEALTH BENEFITS OF JACKFRUIT

Unlike animal sources of protein, jackfruit contains no saturated fat or cholesterol. It is rich in fibre, as well as potassium and iron.

It is important to note that whilst jackfruit is a healthy alternative to meat, the protein contents are relatively low so it is best when paired with beans or pulses for a balanced meal. Or make sure to get more protein from other meals.

Below is a nutritional breakdown based on a can of 'Native Forest – Organic Young Jackfruit' in water:

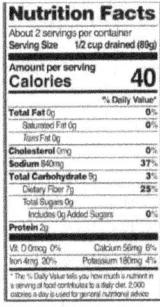

- **Prevents anaemia** - jackfruit seeds are a great source of iron, which is a component of haemoglobin. A diet rich in iron eliminates the risk of anaemia and other blood disorders. Iron also helps to keep the brain and heart healthy and strong.
- **Improves digestion** – young jackfruit in particular, is packed with fibre, which helps improve digestion and prevent constipation. It is also good to help fill you up which may contribute to weight loss. Diets rich in fibre are associated with a reduced risk of developing certain diseases such as heart disease, cancer and type-2 diabetes.
- **Low GI** – a study published in The Ceylon Medical Journal categorised jackfruit as a low-glycaemic index fruit, due to its fibre content. Consumption of young, green jackfruit can even be used to fight high blood sugar levels, according to a Sydney University Glycaemic Index Research Service study.
- **Helps prevent osteoporosis** – a serving of jackfruit contains 6% of your recommended daily allowance of calcium, which helps to reduce the risk of osteoporosis.
- **Less processed** than other vegan meat substitutes such as tofu, tempeh, or seitan.

SUSTAINABLE FOOD SOURCE

Compared to the intensive land and water resources necessary to produce meat, jackfruit is far more efficient as a global food source.

Jackfruit is easy to grow in tropical climates and is resilient against pests, diseases, and high temperatures and is drought-resistant. An interesting use of jackfruit in the years ahead may be to help replace wheat, corn and other staple crops, which are becoming less and less available in Southeast Asia due to climate change (especially rising temperatures and less rain).

Not only is jackfruit a sustainable and ethical meat replacement, it could become an important food source to help world hunger. The perennial trees can grow 100 to 200 fruits in a year, and each fruit can weigh up to 100lbs (45g). As jackfruit is so is rich in calories and nutrients, if a person eats 10 to 12 bulbs, he or she won't need food for another 12 hours.

The jackfruit tree itself is also put to good use as it provides high-quality, rot-resistant timber for furniture and musical instruments. The orange bark can be also be used as dye to make the traditional robes worn by monks. There are so many wonderful uses from this plant!

HOW TO PREPARE

You can go and buy a whole gigantic jackfruit and do all the work of breaking it down yourself, or you can take the easier route and buy it prepared. Besides, it is incredibly difficult to find fresh jackfruit for sale outside of tropical countries, which is probably just as well because they are HUGE.

Jackfruit can be purchased frozen, dried, or canned, either in brine or water for savoury dishes or in syrup for sweet dishes. All the recipes in this book are based on tinned jackfruit in either brine or water. Be careful not to buy the cans in syrup, as they won't work for these recipes. Each tin will have 15-20 pieces of jackfruit inside. You will need to drain them and rinse well, especially if it's in brine, to flush away any salty flavours. After this you can pretty much do what you want with the jackfruit as if it were meat – fry it, bake it, marinade it, etc. Typically, you will begin to shred the pieces after rinsing them. This will break up the fibres so they absorb more of the flavours you are using in the dish. You can shred the pieces with a fork, with your hands, or using a potato masher to get the pulled texture. I find it is easiest pressing down using a fork. However, each recipe will explain the best preparation for the dish. Some people say to cut off and discard the core from the jackfruit pieces, but I think that's a waste. It won't shred like the other pieces, but it still cooks and tastes just as "meaty."

Jackfruit's texture and ability to absorb flavour are it's main selling points - it blows things like tofu out of the water. The trick is to use it with lots of seasoning or sauce to provide flavour and give it plenty of time to absorb it. This means often cooking the jackfruit in spices first, leaving it to marinade in the fridge, or using a slow cooker. Don't try it on its own straight from the can and expect it to taste like chicken breast!

The following recipes will give you a step-by-step guide to best prepare the jackfruit with optional extras such as whether you want to it crispier, or slow-cooked for enhanced flavour and tenderness.

WHERE TO BUY

There doesn't seem to be an easy way to get fresh jackfruit outside of tropical countries. None of the major supermarkets or online organic fruit and veg suppliers seem to stock it.

Most commonly, jackfruit comes in a can and is labelled "young" and "green". Make sure it is in water or brine, NOT in syrup, as this won't work for the recipes in this book.

Here are some of the places you can buy canned jackfruit:

- **In the UK**, major supermarkets such as Sainsbury's, ASDA, Waitrose, and Ocado, are selling it online and in large stores
- **In the USA**, you can find it at Trader Joe's, Whole Foods, and Thrive Market
- **Amazon** sell it in both the UK and the USA (and probably other countries too)
- **Your local Asian, Indian, or Caribbean food stores or online**. Be aware that other names for jackfruit include jaca or chakka (in India), kathal (in Bangladesh), kanun (Thailand), nagka (in Malaysia) or "tree mutton" in Bengali

SUSTAINABLE FOOD SOURCE

Compared to the intensive land and water resources necessary to produce meat, jackfruit is far more efficient as a global food source.

Jackfruit is easy to grow in tropical climates and is resilient against pests, diseases, and high temperatures and is drought-resistant. An interesting use of jackfruit in the years ahead may be to help replace wheat, corn and other staple crops, which are becoming less and less available in Southeast Asia due to climate change (especially rising temperatures and less rain).

Not only is jackfruit a sustainable and ethical meat replacement, it could become an important food source to help world hunger. The perennial trees can grow 100 to 200 fruits in a year, and each fruit can weigh up to 100lbs (45g). As jackfruit is so is rich in calories and nutrients, if a person eats 10 to 12 bulbs, he or she won't need food for another 12 hours.

The jackfruit tree itself is also put to good use as it provides high-quality, rot-resistant timber for furniture and musical instruments. The orange bark can be also be used as dye to make the traditional robes worn by monks. There are so many wonderful uses from this plant!

HOW TO PREPARE

You can go and buy a whole gigantic jackfruit and do all the work of breaking it down yourself, or you can take the easier route and buy it prepared. Besides, it is incredibly difficult to find fresh jackfruit for sale outside of tropical countries, which is probably just as well because they are HUGE.

Jackfruit can be purchased frozen, dried, or canned, either in brine or water for savoury dishes or in syrup for sweet dishes. All the recipes in this book are based on tinned jackfruit in either brine or water. Be careful not to buy the cans in syrup, as they won't work for these recipes.

Each tin will have 15-20 pieces of jackfruit inside. You will need to drain them and rinse well, especially if it's in brine, to flush away any salty flavours. After this you can pretty much do what you want with the jackfruit as if it were meat – fry it, bake it, marinade it, etc. Typically, you will begin to shred the pieces after rinsing them. This will break up the fibres so they absorb more of the flavours you are using in the dish. You can shred the pieces with a fork, with your hands, or using a potato masher to get the pulled texture. I find it is easiest pressing down using a fork. However, each recipe will explain the best preparation for the dish. Some people say to cut off and discard the core from the jackfruit pieces, but I think that's a waste. It won't shred like the other pieces, but it still cooks and tastes just as "meaty."

Jackfruit's texture and ability to absorb flavour are it's main selling points - it blows things like tofu out of the water. The trick is to use it with lots of seasoning or sauce to provide flavour and give it plenty of time to absorb it. This means often cooking the jackfruit in spices first, leaving it to marinade in the fridge, or using a slow cooker. Don't try it on its own straight from the can and expect it to taste like chicken breast!

The following recipes will give you a step-by-step guide to best prepare the jackfruit with optional extras such as whether you want to it crispier, or slow-cooked for enhanced flavour and tenderness.

WHERE TO BUY

There doesn't seem to be an easy way to get fresh jackfruit outside of tropical countries. None of the major supermarkets or online organic fruit and veg suppliers seem to stock it.

Most commonly, jackfruit comes in a can and is labelled "young" and "green". Make sure it is in water or brine, NOT in syrup, as this won't work for the recipes in this book.

Here are some of the places you can buy canned jackfruit:
- **In the UK**, major supermarkets such as Sainsbury's, ASDA, Waitrose, and Ocado, are selling it online and in large stores
- **In the USA**, you can find it at Trader Joe's, Whole Foods, and Thrive Market
- **Amazon** sell it in both the UK and the USA (and probably other countries too)
- **Your local Asian, Indian, or Caribbean food stores or online**. Be aware that other names for jackfruit include jaca or chakka (in India), kathal (in Bangladesh), kanun (Thailand), nagka (in Malaysia) or "tree mutton" in Bengali

HEALTH BENEFITS OF JACKFRUIT

Unlike animal sources of protein, jackfruit contains no saturated fat or cholesterol. It is rich in fibre, as well as potassium and iron.

It is important to note that whilst jackfruit is a healthy alternative to meat, the protein contents are relatively low so it is best when paired with beans or pulses for a balanced meal. Or make sure to get more protein from other meals.

Below is a nutritional breakdown based on a can of 'Native Forest – Organic Young Jackfruit' in water:

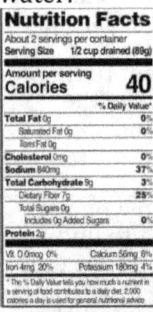

- **Prevents anaemia** - jackfruit seeds are a great source of iron, which is a component of haemoglobin. A diet rich in iron eliminates the risk of anaemia and other blood disorders. Iron also helps to keep the brain and heart healthy and strong.
- **Improves digestion** – young jackfruit in particular, is packed with fibre, which helps improve digestion and prevent constipation. It is also good to help fill you up which may contribute to weight loss. Diets rich in fibre are associated with a reduced risk of developing certain diseases such as heart disease, cancer and type-2 diabetes.
- **Low GI** – a study published in The Ceylon Medical Journal categorised jackfruit as a low-glycaemic index fruit, due to its fibre content. Consumption of young, green jackfruit can even be used to fight high blood sugar levels, according to a Sydney University Glycaemic Index Research Service study.
- **Helps prevent osteoporosis** – a serving of jackfruit contains 6% of your recommended daily allowance of calcium, which helps to reduce the risk of osteoporosis.
- **Less processed** than other vegan meat substitutes such as tofu, tempeh, or seitan.

RECIPES
CHICK'N & SWEET CORN SOUP

SERVES 6 AS A SMALL STARTER OR SIDE
2 x 400g tins of young, green jackfruit in water/brine
1 x 400g tin of creamed corn
150g sweet corn, drained (1-2 tins depending on size)
2 celery stalks, roughly chopped (keep the leaves for garnish)
4 spring onions, thinly sliced (save some for garnish)
½ onion, diced
juice of 1 lemon
1 thumb-sized piece of ginger, peeled and chopped
3 garlic cloves, minced
4 vegetable stock cubes
1 tablespoon tamari
1½ teaspoons chilli powder
1 teaspoon turmeric powder
vegetable oil

This Chinese favourite is a satisfying winter warmer to enjoy on its own or as a starter before a main such as our Peking Jack pancakes on page 34.

Drain and rinse the jackfruit pieces under cold water. Squeeze as much liquid out of the jackfruit flesh as possible. Set aside.

In a large saucepan over a medium heat, pour a tablespoon of vegetable oil. Once hot, throw in the chopped spring onion, onion, celery, and sweet corn kernels.

Fry for 3 to 5 minutes before adding in the prepared jackfruit along with the minced garlic, ginger, and chilli flakes. Cook for a further 10 minutes, stirring frequently until soft and fragrant. Add in 1 litre of boiling water, the vegetable stock cubes, turmeric and lemon juice.

Bring to a boil for 10 minutes before adding in the tamari and creamed corn. Stir through, then taste and adjust with more seasoning if required. You can break up the jackfruit pieces to be 'more stringy' with a fork at this point if you want.

Reduce to a simmer for a further 10 minutes. Serve immediately and decorate with chopped spring onion and celery leaves on top.

HOT & SOUR WONTON SOUP

SERVES 4

FOR THE WONTONS

1 x 400g tin young, green jackfruit in water/brine
1 small sweet potato, finely chopped
1 red bell pepper, finely chopped
40g finely chopped shiitake mushrooms
1 garlic clove, minced
1 thumb-sized piece of ginger, peeled and chopped
1 tablespoon tamari
1 tablespoon almond butter
1 tablespoon rice vinegar
1 teaspoon chilli flakes
1 tablespoon vegetable oil
18-20 vegan wonton wrappers

FOR THE BROTH

500ml water
2 tablespoons tamari
1 tablespoon lime juice
1 tablespoon rice vinegar
1 tablespoon sesame oil
2 tablespoons chilli oil
1 teaspoon maple syrup
1 tablespoon chopped spring onions for garnish

Juicy jackfruit meets hot and sour in this bowl of goodness. Once you've made your own wontons, you won't look back.

Heat the vegetable oil in a large pan over a medium heat. Add the minced garlic and ginger and cook for 2 minutes until fragrant.

Add in the chopped sweet potato, red bell pepper, and shiitake mushrooms, and cook for around 8 minutes or until soft. Stir regularly to make sure the vegetables don't stick to the bottom of the pan.

Drain and rinse the jackfruit. Use a fork or potato masher to break it up so it has a texture similar to pulled pork. Tip the jackfruit in to the pan and cook for 2-3 minutes, stirring regularly. Pour in the tamari, rice vinegar, almond butter, and chilli flakes. Stir well to combine so all the jackfruit pieces are coated and cook for one more minute. Remove from the heat and leave to cool.

Bring a large pot of water to boil. Meanwhile, start preparing the wontons. Place a wonton wrapper on a chopping board. Using your index finger slightly wet the edges with cold water. Place 2 teaspoons of the jackfruit filling in the middle of the wrapper. Fold the wrapper in half over the filling to form a triangle, press down the edges to seal. Make sure to give it a good pinch so that it's fully sealed and won't fall apart during cooking (this is important!). Moisten one bottom corner of the triangle with water. Bring together the left and right corners as if it were hugging itself and press to seal. Repeat with the remaining wrappers and filling.

Once your wontons are ready and the water is boiling, carefully drop the wontons into the boiling water. Lower the heat to simmer, and cook for 2 minutes.

Prepare the broth by combining all the ingredients except the spring onions in a saucepan. Place over a medium heat for 3-5 minutes then pour into 4 bowls. Drain the wontons and place in the bowls with the hot broth. Top with the spring onion and chilli flakes.

CHICK'N NOODLE SOUP

SERVES 6

1 x 400g tin young green jackfruit in water/brine
1 onion, roughly chopped
3 celery stalks, roughly chopped
2 large carrots, roughly chopped
1 garlic clove, minced
pinch of black pepper
2 litres (8 cups) vegetable stock
12oz egg-free wide noodles
1 bay leaf
teaspoon chopped parsley
1 tablespoon vegetable oil

Whenever I think of this dish, that scene from Friends where Joey keeps saying, "Mmm noodle soup" always pops into my head! Anyway, it's a nourishing bowl of goodness to soothe the soul and my go-to dish whenever I start to feel like I'm getting sick.

Heat a tablespoon of oil in a large pot over a medium heat. Add the chopped onion, celery, carrots, garlic and black pepper and cook for 5-8 minutes or until soft.

Meanwhile, boil the kettle to make the vegetable stock.

Drain and rinse the jackfruit, then shred the pieces with a fork before adding to the pot, along with the vegetable stock and bay leaf.

Bring to a boil then reduce to simmer for 20-30 minutes.

Turn the heat back up so the bubbles are closer to boiling. Add the noodles for 8-10 minutes and serve immediately with a sprinkling of fresh parsley.

TIP: If you want to make extra to freeze, omit adding the noodles otherwise they will go mushy when reheated. They can be cooked in a separate pan and then added to the jackfruit soup.

GOULASH SOUP

SERVES 4
FOR THE GOULASH
1 x 400g tin young green jackfruit in water/brine
1 x 400g tin chopped tomatoes
1 x 400g tin chickpeas
1 onion, sliced
2 red bell peppers, chopped
4 tablespoons vegetable oil
2 garlic cloves, finely chopped
2 tablespoons tomato purée
1 tablespoon caraway seeds
1 tablespoon dried oregano
400ml vegetable stock
pinch of cayenne pepper, plus extra to taste
1 tablespoon plain flour
2 tablespoons sweet paprika
salt and pepper

FOR THE MASHED POTATO
6-8 medium Yukon gold potatoes, cut into large chunks
4 tablespoons vegan butter
salt and pepper

Goulash is kind of in between a soup and stew. Nevertheless, it's a hearty and warming meal in a bowl to get you through cold winter days. The jackfruit mops up the flavours beautifully to imitate beef from the Hungarian classic. Make sure to get Yukon potatoes for the mash to get the best fluffy consistency.

In a large saucepan, heat half the oil (2 tablespoons) over a low-medium heat then add the onion and peppers and cook for 15 minutes until softened.

Add the garlic, tomato purée, caraway seeds and oregano and cook for a further two minutes, then tip in the canned tomatoes, drained chickpeas and vegetable stock. Season with salt and pepper and a small pinch of cayenne pepper.

Reduce the heat to a simmer and cook with a lid on for 20 minutes. Add a splash more water if the mixture looks as though it is drying out or thickening too much.

Meanwhile, drain the jackfruit, rinse under colder water, then season with some black pepper. Mix the flour and paprika in a shallow bowl, coat the jackfruit chunks, and shake away any excess flour.

Heat the remaining oil in a frying pan. Add the coated jackfruit and fry over medium-high heat until nicely browned on all sides. Add to the goulash mix with any of the remaining flour and paprika mix. The goulash should still have 25-30 minutes left to cook, so let it simmer away. If the mixture still looks too thick, you can add a splash more water here.

Whilst this is cooking, prepare the mashed potatoes. Place the potatoes in a large pan of boiling water with some salt and cook for around 20 minutes until a fork easily glides through the potato.

Drain the potatoes then transfer back to the empty pan to mash with a potato masher until fluffy. Add the vegan butter, salt and pepper, and combine.

When the goulash is ready, taste and add more seasoning or cayenne if needed. Serve with a dollop of creamy mashed potatoes or alternatively a piece of crusty bread.

GOULASH SOUP

SERVES 4
FOR THE GOULASH
1 x 400g tin young green jackfruit in water/brine
1 x 400g tin chopped tomatoes
1 x 400g tin chickpeas
1 onion, sliced
2 red bell peppers, chopped
4 tablespoons vegetable oil
2 garlic cloves, finely chopped
2 tablespoons tomato purée
1 tablespoon caraway seeds
1 tablespoon dried oregano
400ml vegetable stock
pinch of cayenne pepper, plus extra to taste
1 tablespoon plain flour
2 tablespoons sweet paprika
salt and pepper

FOR THE MASHED POTATO
6-8 medium Yukon gold potatoes, cut into large chunks
4 tablespoons vegan butter
salt and pepper

Goulash is kind of in between a soup and stew. Nevertheless, it's a hearty and warming meal in a bowl to get you through cold winter days. The jackfruit mops up the flavours beautifully to imitate beef from the Hungarian classic. Make sure to get Yukon potatoes for the mash to get the best fluffy consistency.

In a large saucepan, heat half the oil (2 tablespoons) over a low-medium heat then add the onion and peppers and cook for 15 minutes until softened.

Add the garlic, tomato purée, caraway seeds and oregano and cook for a further two minutes, then tip in the canned tomatoes, drained chickpeas and vegetable stock. Season with salt and pepper and a small pinch of cayenne pepper.

Reduce the heat to a simmer and cook with a lid on for 20 minutes. Add a splash more water if the mixture looks as though it is drying out or thickening too much.

Meanwhile, drain the jackfruit, rinse under colder water, then season with some black pepper. Mix the flour and paprika in a shallow bowl, coat the jackfruit chunks, and shake away any excess flour.

Heat the remaining oil in a frying pan. Add the coated jackfruit and fry over medium-high heat until nicely browned on all sides. Add to the goulash mix with any of the remaining flour and paprika mix. The goulash should still have 25-30 minutes left to cook, so let it simmer away. If the mixture still looks too thick, you can add a splash more water here.

Whilst this is cooking, prepare the mashed potatoes. Place the potatoes in a large pan of boiling water with some salt and cook for around 20 minutes until a fork easily glides through the potato.

Drain the potatoes then transfer back to the empty pan to mash with a potato masher until fluffy. Add the vegan butter, salt and pepper, and combine.

When the goulash is ready, taste and add more seasoning or cayenne if needed. Serve with a dollop of creamy mashed potatoes or alternatively a piece of crusty bread.

CHICK'N NOODLE SOUP

SERVES 6

1 x 400g tin young green jackfruit in water/brine
1 onion, roughly chopped
3 celery stalks, roughly chopped
2 large carrots, roughly chopped
1 garlic clove, minced
pinch of black pepper
2 litres (8 cups) vegetable stock
12oz egg-free wide noodles
1 bay leaf
teaspoon chopped parsley
1 tablespoon vegetable oil

Whenever I think of this dish, that scene from Friends where Joey keeps saying, "Mmm noodle soup" always pops into my head! Anyway, it's a nourishing bowl of goodness to soothe the soul and my go-to dish whenever I start to feel like I'm getting sick.

Heat a tablespoon of oil in a large pot over a medium heat. Add the chopped onion, celery, carrots, garlic and black pepper and cook for 5-8 minutes or until soft.

Meanwhile, boil the kettle to make the vegetable stock.

Drain and rinse the jackfruit, then shred the pieces with a fork before adding to the pot, along with the vegetable stock and bay leaf.

Bring to a boil then reduce to simmer for 20-30 minutes.

Turn the heat back up so the bubbles are closer to boiling. Add the noodles for 8-10 minutes and serve immediately with a sprinkling of fresh parsley.

TIP: If you want to make extra to freeze, omit adding the noodles otherwise they will go mushy when reheated. They can be cooked in a separate pan and then added to the jackfruit soup.

TOONA MELT SANDWICH

MAKES 2 SANDWICHES
FOR THE TOONA FILLING
1 x 400g tin young green jackfruit in water/brine
1 x 400g can cannellini beans
½ teaspoon olive oil
3 spring onions, chopped
2 garlic cloves, minced
½ teaspoon dried tarragon
6 tablespoons vegenaise
2 tablespoons pickled relish
1 ½ tablespoons vegan Dijon mustard
juice of 1 lemon
salt and pepper
FOR THE SANDWICH
4 slices of bread
handful of grated vegan cheese

Oozy, melty cheese, crispy golden toast, and a toona filling zazzed up with spring onion, garlic, mustard and pickles. Jackfruit does a mighty fine job of stepping in for tuna in this delicious sandwich. Enjoy!

Drain the jackfruit and rinse well. Use a fork to pull apart the jackfruit in to shreds (until it has a tuna-like consistency).

Heat the olive oil in a large frying pan over medium heat. Add the spring onion and garlic and cook for 2-3 minutes until soft. Add the jackfruit cook for 5 minutes, stirring occasionally, until the jackfruit's moisture is gone. Remove from heat to cool.

Meanwhile, use a fork to mash the white beans in a bowl. Once they are thoroughly mashed, add the vegenaise, Dijon mustard, tarragon, pickled relish, and lemon juice. Mix together, then add the jackfruit and mix until it's fully coated. Taste and add seasoning, if necessary.

Turn on the grill of your oven to its highest setting . Layout the 4 slices of bread. Place a small amount of spring onion and tomato on two of the slices of bread. Then top the tomato with the jackfruit mix. On the remaining slices of bread, sprinkle the grated cheese.

Place the two slices of bread, topped with cheese, on a baking sheet and place under the grill. Leave for around 2-4 minutes until the cheese has started to melt.

Remove and place the cheese slices on top of the slices topped with the jackfruit salad. Serve and enjoy!

PHILLY CHEEZESTEAK

MAKES 4 SANDWICHES
2 x 400g tin young green jackfruit in water/brine
2 tablespoons olive oil
1 onion, sliced
½ teaspoon garlic powder
½ teaspoon paprika
½ teaspoon sea salt
¼ teaspoon black pepper
a pinch of cayenne pepper
1 tablespoon chickpea flour
250ml vegetable stock
2 tablespoons vegan Worcestershire sauce
1 tablespoon balsamic vinegar
4 gluten-free rolls
6 tablespoons vegenaise
handful vegan cheese

The undisputed king of the subs, this meaty and gooey vegan version gives you all the feels. Can be served with a side salad or potato wedges if you're feeling indulgent.

Preheat the oven to 200°C (400°F). In a frying pan, heat 1 tablespoon of oil over medium heat. Add the sliced onions and cook for 3 minutes until they start to soften. Reduce the heat to medium-low to caramelise the onions, stirring often. This takes around 10 minutes. Once ready, transfer to a plate and set aside. Leave the pan for reuse.

While the onion is cooking, prepare the jackfruit. Drain and rinse well in water, then chop into small pieces. Place in to a bowl and add the garlic powder, paprika, salt, black pepper, and cayenne pepper. Mix well until the jackfruit is completely coated. Transfer the jackfruit to the frying pan and cook over a medium-high heat for about 5 minutes to lock in the spices.

Add the remaining tablespoon of olive oil to the pan and stir so the jackfruit pieces are evenly coated. Add the caramelised onions back in to the pan and mix with the jackfruit. Add the chickpea flour and mix it well into the oil, onions and jackfruit to help make the gravy. Next, add the vegetable stock, Worcestershire sauce and balsamic vinegar and mix well together.

Lower the heat to medium, cover the pan and leave to simmer for about 15 minutes until the jackfruit is soft and tender. When the jackfruit is soft, use two forks or a potato masher to pull the pieces apart and shred them.

Line a baking tray and transfer the shredded jackfruit in a single layer. Bake for 15 minutes. This will make the jackfruit chewier.

Once you take the jackfruit out, turn the oven grill on to the highest setting. Slice open the bread rolls and spread a thin layer of mayo on each bottom slice. Add the jackfruit on top of these bottom pieces and then top with the shredded cheese. Place the rolls on the baking sheet all facing up. Grill for 2-3 minutes, taking care they don't burn.

Remove from the oven and place the tops of the rolls over the jackfruit. Serve while hot.

THE VEGAN CUBAN

MAKES 2 LARGE SANDWICHES

2 x 400g tins young green jackfruit in water/brine
1 tablespoon of vegan butter
1 tablespoon dried oregano
2 garlic cloves, minced
1 teaspoon cumin
1 teaspoon chilli flakes
1 tablespoon olive oil
2 teaspoons vegan Dijon mustard
1 bunch kale, stalks removed
handful chopped pickles
1 lime (optional)
2 baguettes or sandwich rolls
salt and pepper, to taste

After watching the film Chef I was inspired to try and recreate a vegan version of their famous Cuban sandwich. This is a healthier version but with the fun of a Cuban as you coat and fry the bread in vegan butter (see if you can do it as fast as in the film!).

Preheat the oven to 200°C (400°F).

Drain and rinse the jackfruit. Add the jackfruit to a lined baking tray and spread it out evenly in one layer. Add the minced garlic, oregano, cumin, and olive oil over the jackfruit.

Pop the jackfruit mixture into the oven and cook for 20 minutes.

While it's cooking, rinse your kale and remove the stems. Place a frying pan on medium heat and coat with a splash of olive oil. Place the kale in the pan and cook until it's brown and crispy on each side. Continue until all your pieces have been browned (you may have to do this in batches depending on how big your pan is). Set aside on a plate.

Cut your baguette/bread rolls in half and coat each side with vegan butter. Place each half in your frying pan to toast.

Once your bread is toasted, coat one half with Dijon mustard and the other with pickles.

Remove the jackfruit from the oven and add the chilli flakes, salt, and pepper. Gently work seasonings into the mixture.

Make your sandwiches. Scoop a healthy amount of jackfruit on top of the pickles followed by layers of kale. Serve and enjoy.

SLOW-COOKER REUBEN

MAKES 4 SANDWICHES
FOR THE CORNED JACKFRUIT
1 x 400g tin young green jackfruit in water/brine
juice from 1 x 400g tin of sliced beetroot (reserve beetroot for another use)
1 teaspoon paprika
½ teaspoon mustard powder
1 tablespoon dried thyme
1 tablespoon dried rosemary
salt and pepper
FOR THE SANDWICH FILLING
12 slices gluten-free bread, toasted
8 slices vegan cheese
store-bought sauerkraut (about 6 cups or ¼ cup)
1 tablespoon vegan thousand island dressing
gherkin to serve (optional)

The juice from the beetroots adds a lovely flavour and convincing colour for the corned jackfruit. If you have pickled gherkins handy, I love popping one of these on top of the sandwich with a cocktail stick for presentation.

Drain jackfruit and rinse well. In a medium bowl, shred the jackfruit well with a fork. You may want to cut the hard corner pieces into smaller strips as these don't shred as well.

In a container, add the beetroot juice, paprika, mustard powder, thyme, rosemary, and a pinch of salt and pepper. Mix well to combine. Cover the jackfruit and marinate in the fridge for 1 hour or overnight.

When you're ready to make the sandwiches, drain the jackfruit and place in a large frying pan over a medium heat. Cook for 6-8 minutes.

Place a spoonful of corned jackfruit on to 1 slice of toasted gluten-free bread. Top with a slice of vegan cheese, sauerkraut, and vegan thousand island dressing. Place the other toasted bread on top and cut in to triangles. Secure with a cocktail stick and pop a gherkin on top of the toasted bread. Serve and enjoy.

SLOW-COOKER REUBEN

MAKES 4 SANDWICHES
FOR THE CORNED JACKFRUIT
1 x 400g tin young green jackfruit in water/brine
juice from 1 x 400g tin of sliced beetroot (reserve beetroot for another use)
1 teaspoon paprika
½ teaspoon mustard powder
1 tablespoon dried thyme
1 tablespoon dried rosemary
salt and pepper
FOR THE SANDWICH FILLING
12 slices gluten-free bread, toasted
8 slices vegan cheese
store-bought sauerkraut (about 6 cups or ¼ cup)
1 tablespoon vegan thousand island dressing
gherkin to serve (optional)

The juice from the beetroots adds a lovely flavour and convincing colour for the corned jackfruit. If you have pickled gherkins handy, I love popping one of these on top of the sandwich with a cocktail stick for presentation.

Drain jackfruit and rinse well. In a medium bowl, shred the jackfruit well with a fork. You may want to cut the hard corner pieces into smaller strips as these don't shred as well.

In a container, add the beetroot juice, paprika, mustard powder, thyme, rosemary, and a pinch of salt and pepper. Mix well to combine. Cover the jackfruit and marinate in the fridge for 1 hour or overnight.

When you're ready to make the sandwiches, drain the jackfruit and place in a large frying pan over a medium heat. Cook for 6-8 minutes.

Place a spoonful of corned jackfruit on to 1 slice of toasted gluten-free bread. Top with a slice of vegan cheese, sauerkraut, and vegan thousand island dressing. Place the other toasted bread on top and cut in to triangles. Secure with a cocktail stick and pop a gherkin on top of the toasted bread. Serve and enjoy.

THE VEGAN CUBAN

MAKES 2 LARGE SANDWICHES

2 x 400g tins young green jackfruit in water/brine
1 tablespoon of vegan butter
1 tablespoon dried oregano
2 garlic cloves, minced
1 teaspoon cumin
1 teaspoon chilli flakes
1 tablespoon olive oil
2 teaspoons vegan Dijon mustard
1 bunch kale, stalks removed
handful chopped pickles
1 lime (optional)
2 baguettes or sandwich rolls
salt and pepper, to taste

After watching the film Chef I was inspired to try and recreate a vegan version of their famous Cuban sandwich. This is a healthier version but with the fun of a Cuban as you coat and fry the bread in vegan butter (see if you can do it as fast as in the film!).

Preheat the oven to 200°C (400°F).

Drain and rinse the jackfruit. Add the jackfruit to a lined baking tray and spread it out evenly in one layer. Add the minced garlic, oregano, cumin, and olive oil over the jackfruit.

Pop the jackfruit mixture into the oven and cook for 20 minutes.

While it's cooking, rinse your kale and remove the stems. Place a frying pan on medium heat and coat with a splash of olive oil. Place the kale in the pan and cook until it's brown and crispy on each side. Continue until all your pieces have been browned (you may have to do this in batches depending on how big your pan is). Set aside on a plate.

Cut your baguette/bread rolls in half and coat each side with vegan butter. Place each half in your frying pan to toast.

Once your bread is toasted, coat one half with Dijon mustard and the other with pickles. Remove the jackfruit from the oven and add the chilli flakes, salt, and pepper. Gently work seasonings into the mixture.

Make your sandwiches. Scoop a healthy amount of jackfruit on top of the pickles followed by layers of kale. Serve and enjoy.

CRISPY CHICK'N NUGGETS

MAKES 10-12 NUGGETS
FOR THE NUGGETS
2 x 400g tins young green jackfruit in water/brine
250ml unsweetened almond milk
1-1½ tablespoons apple cider vinegar
255g plain flour
100g corn flour
1 tablespoon baking powder
salt and pepper
1 tablespoon vegetable oil
1 teaspoon hot sauce (optional)
FOR THE DIPPING SAUCE
6 tablespoons vegenaise
2-3 tablespoons English mustard
2 tablespoons agave nectar

This recipe took a few revisions to get the crunchiness right but oh my, these nuggets are so moreish! We've even had our non-vegan friends munching on them and coming back for more.
Start by making the dipping sauce. Mix the vegenaise, mustard, and agave nectar in a bowl. Set aside or in the fridge whilst you make the nuggets.
Next, drain and rinse the jackfruit pieces taking care not to break them up.
Combine the almond milk with the apple cider vinegar for the 'buttermilk'. Add the jackfruit pieces and mix so all sides are covered. Set aside.
Meanwhile, whisk together the flour, corn flour, and baking powder for the batter.
Heat the vegetable oil in a saucepan over a medium heat. To check if it's hot enough, test with a pinch of flour and if it sizzles, it's ready.
Take a few pieces of jackfruit at a time from the 'buttermilk' mixture and drop in the flour. Turn each piece so it's covered on all sides. Quickly coat in the buttermilk again and then coat again in the flour mixture (this is what gives it the extra crispiness!).
Gently place the pieces into the oil. Toss occasionally and remove with a strainer when golden brown to paper towels to drain any excess oil. Serve immediately with the dipping sauce.

BBQ PULLED-NOT-PORK BURGER

MAKES 6 BURGERS

2 x 400g tins young, green jackfruit in water/brine
1 onion, diced
3 garlic cloves, minced
6 tablespoons BBQ sauce
1 teaspoon smoked paprika
½ teaspoon garlic powder
½ teaspoon onion powder
50ml water
salt and pepper
tablespoon olive oil
6 whole-wheat hamburger buns
optional toppings: lettuce, pineapple, cabbage slaw, avocado

This was one of the very first jackfruit recipes I made and it's one I regularly come back to as it's so delicious! My favourite is adding some slaw as a topping and serving alongside some sweet potato fries.

Drain and thoroughly rinse the jackfruit.

Heat one tablespoon olive oil in a frying pan over a medium heat. Add the chopped onion and garlic and cook for 5-7 minutes until soft.

Add the jackfruit, BBQ sauce, and 50ml water. Stir and cover. Turn the heat down to medium-low.

Cook for 15 minutes, then stir again, adding more water if needed. Cover and cook for another 15 minutes.

Using a potato masher or a fork, shred the jackfruit until it resembles pulled pork. Add the smoked paprika, garlic powder, onion powder, salt and pepper. Stir to combine and add more BBQ sauce if desired.

Spoon the pulled jackfruit mix in to the burger buns and serve with toppings of your choice.

SMOKY CHICK'N SALAD

SERVES 4

1 x 400g tin young, green jackfruit in water/brine
2 celery stalks, finely chopped
3 spring onions, thinly sliced
1 red bell pepper, chopped
3 tablespoons vegenaise
1 garlic clove, minced
3 teaspoons fresh dill, finely chopped
3 teaspoons lemon juice, to taste
½ teaspoon smoked paprika
salt and pepper

Easy to whip up on a summer's evening for a light dinner, or to take along to a picnic. Sometimes if I'm feeling indulgent, I make some croutons to go on top, or serve with some smashed avocado.

Drain and rinse the jackfruit. Place the jackfruit pieces on a chopping board and shred with a fork so that they resemble pulled pork.

Add the jackfruit pieces to a bowl and stir in the chopped celery, spring onions, red bell pepper, vegenaise, and minced garlic until combined.

Now stir in the dill and season with the lemon juice, smoked paprika, salt, and pepper. Taste after mixing and adjust seasoning quantities if needed.

Serve in a sandwich or wrap on a bed of lettuce. I love adding croutons and smashed avocado to go all out for a big salad. Leftovers can be refrigerated in an airtight container for 3 to 4 days.

TOONA COLLARD WRAPS

SERVES 4

1 x 400g tin young, green jackfruit in water/brine
4 large collard wraps
6 tablespoons hummus
200g cherry tomatoes, chopped
½ red or yellow bell pepper, chopped
2 spring onions, sliced
1 cucumber, sliced
150g quinoa
salt and pepper
2 tablespoons vegenaise (optional)

Light and refreshing, perfect for a summer lunch. I find they are good for meal prep as they last in the fridge for 2-3 days in an airtight container and the jackfruit absorbs even more flavour.

Fill a medium saucepan with 300ml water (it should be about double the volume of your quinoa) and bring to the boil.

Once the water is boiling, add the rinsed quinoa. Cover and reduce heat to simmer. Cook for approximately 25 minutes until the quinoa is soft and the water has been completely absorbed.

Meanwhile, chop the cherry tomatoes, bell pepper, spring onion, and cucumber into small pieces so they can be easily rolled in a wrap.

Rinse and drain the jackfruit. Add to a bowl and at this point you can mix with vegenaise if you prefer. You can also choose to skip this step and simply mix jackfruit in a bowl without adding any additional condiments.

Next, take a large frying pan and add 300ml water. Remove the pan from heat once the water is boiling and quickly blanch each collard wrap by submerging them from 3 seconds in the water. This is so the collard wraps become much softer and easier to wrap.

Once the quinoa is cooked, remove from the heat and begin to assemble your collard wraps. Begin by layering hummus, quinoa, and vegetables. Finish your collard wraps by adding a layer of jackfruit, and then topping with sea salt and pepper to taste.

To roll your collard wraps simply fold in each side and then roll from the bottom up. Serve and enjoy.

VEGAN QUICHE LORRAINE

MAKES 1 LARGE QUICHE OR 4 SMALL QUICHES
2 x 400g tins young, green jackfruit in water/brine
1 tablespoon olive oil
1 large onion, finely chopped
1 medium chilli, thinly sliced and seeds removed
1 box (349g) firm silken tofu
½ lemon
2 tablespoons nutritional yeast
1 tablespoon tahini
4 tablespoons almond milk
salt and pepper
short crust pastry
fresh parsley, to garnish (optional)

I made this once for a Christmas party buffet with people not believing it was vegan, as it tastes so good! If you have more than one quiche tin, it's great to make more than one at a time as they keep in the fridge as a nice leftovers lunch.

Preheat the oven to 200°C (400°F).

Line 4 mini quiche tins or one large quiche tin with greaseproof paper or oil. Line the tins with the short crust pastry and trim off any excess. Prick the bottom of the cases and bake them for around five minutes. Remove from the oven and set aside.

In a large pan, add a tablespoon olive oil on medium heat. Add the chopped onion and cook for 5-8 minutes until golden, stirring frequently.

Add in the chopped chilli and fry for a further 3-5 minutes until soft.

Drain and rinse the jackfruit. Add the pieces to the pan and fry for a further 5 minutes.

Meanwhile, in a food processor/blender, add in the silken tofu, lemon juice, nutritional yeast, tahini, almond milk, and salt and pepper. Whizz up until smooth and creamy.

Fold the jackfruit mixture into the tofu mixture to combine.

Fill the pastry cases with the quiche filling. Pop the quiches back in to the oven and cook for around 15 minutes.

The quiches can be enjoyed warm straight from the oven or cold with a salad. Top with a few pieces of fresh parsley for garnish. Quiches can be stored in a sealed container in the fridge for up to 2 days.

VIETNAMESE SALAD

SERVES 2
FOR THE SALAD
1 x 400g tin young, green jackfruit in water/brine
1 tablespoon toasted sesame seeds
1 tablespoon vegetable oil
100g oyster mushrooms, finely chopped
½ medium carrot, cut into matchstick pieces
½ small onion, thinly sliced.
handful coriander, roughly chopped
handful mint, roughly chopped
salt and pepper
FOR THE DRESSING
3 tablespoons sugar
¼ cup water
2 tablespoons rice vinegar
1 teaspoon soy sauce
1 tablespoon lime juice.
½ red chilli, seeded and finely chopped
1 garlic clove, finely chopped
pinch of salt

Sweet, tangy, crunchy – this salad is packed with flavour. It goes perfectly with a glass of cold white wine on a summer's day.

Prepare the toasted sesame seeds in a frying pan on medium heat for a couple of minutes until they start to turn brown. Set aside.

Drain and rinse the jackfruit. Shred the pieces with a fork and set aside in a large bowl.

Heat the olive oil in a large frying pan over a medium-high heat. Add the oyster mushrooms, a pinch of salt and pepper, stirring to coat the mushrooms lightly with oil. Cook for 3-5 minutes to brown the mushrooms.

Push the jackfruit to one side of the bowl and spoon the mushrooms in to the empty side to cool. Add the chopped carrot, onion, coriander, and mint over the jackfruit and mix together.

Pour the dressing ingredients in to a bowl and mix well. Scoop the salad with your hands or a slotted spoon, leaving most of the dressing in the bowl, onto a serving dish. Serve the remaining dressing back over the salad or in a side dish, to taste.

Decoratively sprinkle the toasted sesame seeds over the top.

NICOISE SALAD

SERVES 4
FOR THE SALAD
1 x 400g tins young, green jackfruit in water/brine
250g cherry tomatoes
200g green beans, roughly chopped
½ onion, sliced
500g baby new potatoes, chopped in half
2 sweet gem lettuce
2 celery sticks
100g black olives
FOR THE DRESSING
1 tablespoon capers, drained
2 tablespoons vegan Dijon mustard
2 tablespoons white wine vinegar
6 tablespoons olive oil (extra virgin if possible)
lemon juice, to taste
salt and pepper

This salty, mustardy dressing gets quickly soaked up by the jackfruit to imitate tuna in this classic salad. Don't be too precious with the salad quantities, I tend to just grab a handful of the vegetables per portion I'm making.

Put a saucepan filled with lightly salted water on a high heat and bring to a boil. Add the new potatoes and turn down to simmer for 10 minutes. Drain and set to one side to cool.

Meanwhile, mix together all the ingredients for the dressing, tasting and adjusting for more seasoning or lemon juice if desired.

Drain the jackfruit and rinse well under water. In a large bowl, break up the gem lettuce and add the cherry tomatoes, green beans, celery, onion, black olives, and jackfruit. Add the new potatoes once they have cooled.

Lightly dress the salad and mix well. Serve and enjoy

SLOW-COOKER CHILLI

SERVES 8

1 x 400g tin young, green jackfruit in water/brine
1 onion, chopped
1 red bell pepper, chopped
2 x 400g tins chopped tomatoes
2 tablespoons tomato purée
1 green chilli, sliced and seeds removed
1 x 400g tin black beans
juice of one lime
1 teaspoon oregano
1 teaspoon chilli powder
1 teaspoon smoked paprika
2 teaspoon cumin
1 tablespoon maple syrup
olive oil
salt and pepper

If I had to choose a favourite recipe for this book, this would be it. When slow-cooked, the flavours in this chilli are to die for. Make a big batch as it freezes well and can be served in so many different ways. I hope you love it as much as I do.

Rinse and drain jackfruit. Pull the pieces apart with a fork to resemble pulled pork.

Put a frying pan over a medium heat and add a tablespoon of olive oil. Add the onions and chopped chilli and cook for 3-5 minutes until the onion is soft.

Add the jackfruit to the pan and season with the oregano, chilli powder, smoked paprika, and cumin. Cook for a further 5 minutes, stirring to ensure the jackfruit is evenly covered.

Take the pan off the heat and transfer contents to a crockpot or slow cooker. Drain the black beans and rinse, then add to the crockpot, followed by the chopped tomatoes. Throw in the chopped bell pepper, squeeze of maple syrup, lime juice, and tomato purée. Season with salt and pepper, then mix well so the ingredients are evenly distributed.

Cook on high for 2-3 hours or on low for 5-6 hours.

Serve with fluffy basmati rice. Alternative sides include tortilla chips, homemade guacamole, grated vegan cheese, and vegan soured cream.

SLOW-COOKER CHILLI

SERVES 8

1 x 400g tin young, green jackfruit in water/brine
1 onion, chopped
1 red bell pepper, chopped
2 x 400g tins chopped tomatoes
2 tablespoons tomato purée
1 green chilli, sliced and seeds removed
1 x 400g tin black beans
juice of one lime
1 teaspoon oregano
1 teaspoon chilli powder
1 teaspoon smoked paprika
2 teaspoon cumin
1 tablespoon maple syrup
olive oil
salt and pepper

If I had to choose a favourite recipe for this book, this would be it. When slow-cooked, the flavours in this chilli are to die for. Make a big batch as it freezes well and can be served in so many different ways. I hope you love it as much as I do.

Rinse and drain jackfruit. Pull the pieces apart with a fork to resemble pulled pork.

Put a frying pan over a medium heat and add a tablespoon of olive oil. Add the onions and chopped chilli and cook for 3-5 minutes until the onion is soft.

Add the jackfruit to the pan and season with the oregano, chilli powder, smoked paprika, and cumin. Cook for a further 5 minutes, stirring to ensure the jackfruit is evenly covered.

Take the pan off the heat and transfer contents to a crockpot or slow cooker. Drain the black beans and rinse, then add to the crockpot, followed by the chopped tomatoes. Throw in the chopped bell pepper, squeeze of maple syrup, lime juice, and tomato purée. Season with salt and pepper, then mix well so the ingredients are evenly distributed.

Cook on high for 2-3 hours or on low for 5-6 hours.

Serve with fluffy basmati rice. Alternative sides include tortilla chips, homemade guacamole, grated vegan cheese, and vegan soured cream.

NICOISE SALAD

SERVES 4
FOR THE SALAD
1 x 400g tins young, green jackfruit in water/brine
250g cherry tomatoes
200g green beans, roughly chopped
½ onion, sliced
500g baby new potatoes, chopped in half
2 sweet gem lettuce
2 celery sticks
100g black olives
FOR THE DRESSING
1 tablespoon capers, drained
2 tablespoons vegan Dijon mustard
2 tablespoons white wine vinegar
6 tablespoons olive oil (extra virgin if possible)
lemon juice, to taste
salt and pepper

This salty, mustardy dressing gets quickly soaked up by the jackfruit to imitate tuna in this classic salad. Don't be too precious with the salad quantities, I tend to just grab a handful of the vegetables per portion I'm making.

Put a saucepan filled with lightly salted water on a high heat and bring to a boil. Add the new potatoes and turn down to simmer for 10 minutes. Drain and set to one side to cool.

Meanwhile, mix together all the ingredients for the dressing, tasting and adjusting for more seasoning or lemon juice if desired.

Drain the jackfruit and rinse well under water. In a large bowl, break up the gem lettuce and add the cherry tomatoes, green beans, celery, onion, black olives, and jackfruit. Add the new potatoes once they have cooled.

Lightly dress the salad and mix well. Serve and enjoy

BBQ PULLED-NOT-PORK TACOS

MAKES 10-12 TACOS
FOR THE FILLING
2 x 400g tins young, green jackfruit in water/brine
2 tablespoons extra virgin olive oil
1 small onion, finely chopped
2 cloves garlic, minced
1 red chilli, finely chopped and seeds removed
250ml BBQ sauce
2 teaspoons ground cumin
1 teaspoon dried oregano
1 teaspoon ground coriander
1 teaspoon smoked paprika
salt and pepper

FOR THE TACOS
10-12 small corn tortillas
1 ripe avocado, thinly sliced
handful coriander leaves, roughly chopped
1 lime, cut into wedges
vegan soured cream

I first made these a few years ago and they were incredible. Now they're popping up in shops all over the UK as Christmas appetisers or ready-meals so they must be hitting the spot for other people too! Get creative with the toppings with things like sweet corn, radish, and jalapeños - whatever tickles your pickle.

Rinse and drain the jackfruit. Break apart using a fork into shredded pieces to resemble pulled pork.

Put a large saucepan over a medium heat and add the olive oil. When the oil is hot, add the onion and chilli and cook for 5 minutes. Add the garlic and cook for a further 2 minutes until fragrant, stirring often.

Add the shredded jackfruit to the pan and stir well. Then add the BBQ sauce, cumin, oregano, coriander, smoked paprika and a pinch of salt.

Stir so the jackfruit is evenly coated in the spices and cook for another 4 to 5 minutes. The jackfruit should have browned and be slightly crisped around the edges.

Finally, assemble the tacos. Warm the tortillas and add a large spoonful of cooked jackfruit in the middle of each. Top with avocado, coriander, vegan soured cream and a squeeze of lime

MAC 'N' CHEEZE

SERVES 4

1 x 400g tin young, green jackfruit in water/brine
250ml BBQ sauce
250g macaroni pasta
1 medium-sized sweet potato cooked and peeled
3 tablespoons raw cashews soaked in water overnight
1 garlic clove, minced
250ml unsweetened almond milk
1 tablespoon lemon juice
½ tablespoon soy sauce
¼ teaspoon smoked paprika
¼ teaspoon cayenne pepper
¼ teaspoon mustard powder
2 tablespoons nutritional yeast
1 tablespoon corn flour
salt and pepper

Mac 'n' cheese is the ultimate comfort food. When I used to eat meat I would go crazy for versions with pulled pork or beef in them so once I'd mastered the 'cheeze' vegan version and later discovered the magical jackfruit, I knew this would be another winner.

Soak the cashews overnight.

Cook the sweet potato pieces in a pan of boiling water for 15 minutes. Drain and set aside. Preheat the oven to 200°C (400°F).

Meanwhile, prepare the jackfruit. Drain and rinse well. Using a fork, break up the pieces so they look shredded. Add the jackfruit to a small frying pan and add enough BBQ sauce to coat. Cook on medium heat for 10 minutes, stirring occasionally.

Spread the jackfruit out on a baking sheet and bake for 10 minutes or until it starts to dry out and crisp up. Remove and set aside.

Put a saucepan of water on to boil with some salt. Once boiling, add the macaroni pasta and cook for 10 minutes until al-dente.

Meanwhile, add the sweet potato, cashews, garlic, and a few splashes of almond milk to a blender or food processor. Blend until completely smooth. Add the lemon juice, soy sauce, smoked paprika, cayenne pepper, mustard powder, nutritional yeast, and corn starch. Blend again for a few seconds until combined. Taste for seasoning and adjust as needed.

Transfer the mixture to a saucepan and cook over medium heat, stirring frequently, until it thickens slightly for 2-3 minutes. Fold in the cooked pasta and cook for another 1-2 minutes. Serve topped with BBQ jackfruit.

TOONA PASTA BAKE

SERVES 4

1 x 400g tins young, green jackfruit in water/brine
1 tablespoon olive oil
2 teaspoons onion powder
2 teaspoons garlic powder
salt and pepper
150g penne pasta
1 x 400g tin coconut milk
1 tablespoon corn flour
170g nutritional yeast
1 x 325g sweet corn (260g drained)
170g dry breadcrumbs

When I was little, my brother and I would often go to our neighbour's house for dinner if my parents were working late. For some reason they always cooked tuna pasta bake, so I have very fond childhood memories of this dish. I was delighted when I was able to closely recreate it for my husband as a vegan version.

Preheat your oven to 180°C (350°F).

Prepare a small baking dish. Drain the jackfruit, rinse well and break up into stringy pieces with a fork.

Heat the olive oil in a frying pan and add the jackfruit, along with 1 teaspoon onion powder, 1 teaspoon garlic powder, and a good seasoning with salt and pepper. Cook until the edges begin to brown and the jackfruit is soft. Set aside.

Next cook the pasta by filling a saucepan with lightly salted water and bring to the boil. Add the pasta and cook for 10 minutes until al dente. Drain and set aside.

Using the same saucepan over a medium heat, add the coconut milk, remaining onion powder, garlic powder, salt, pepper, nutritional yeast and corn flour. Whisk constantly over the heat until the sauce thickens.

Add the sweet corn, jackfruit and pasta to the sauce and mix well. Pour the mixture into the baking tray and spread out evenly. Sprinkle the top with breadcrumbs.

Bake in the oven for 20-30 minutes or until golden brown on top. Serve immediately.

HAWAIIAN PIZZA

SERVES 4

2 x 400g tins young, green jackfruit in water/brine
250ml BBQ sauce
2 tablespoons tomato purée
1 tablespoon hot sauce
½ teaspoon smoked paprika
1 tablespoon olive oil
salt and pepper
½ red onion, chopped
2-3 cloves garlic, minced
8 sun-dried tomatoes, chopped
260g pineapple chunks
1 vegan pizza base

Pineapple on a pizza is one of those things you either love or you hate. Obviously I love it, hence this recipe. It goes oh so well with the BBQ pulled jackfruit and I can't wait for you to try it if you're in the pineapple on pizzas camp too.

Preheat your oven to 200°C (400°F).

Drain and rinse the jackfruit and use a fork to tear into shreds. Set aside.

In a small bowl combine the BBQ sauce, hot sauce, tomato purée, smoked paprika, and salt and pepper. Mix and then set aside.

Heat 1 tablespoon of olive oil in a frying pan over medium heat for about 1 minute. Add the chopped onion and garlic, and cook for 3-5 minutes until soft.

Add the jackfruit and cook for a further 5 minutes until most of the liquid from jackfruit has gone.

Add the sauce mixture to the jackfruit in the pan, lower the heat to medium-low, cover and leave for about 10-20 minutes, stirring occasionally. Mix in the sun-dried tomatoes and cook for another 2-3 minutes.

Place the pizza dough on a prepared baking tray and spread the jackfruit mixture out evenly. Top with the pineapple chunks and bake for 10-15 minutes in the oven until the crust turns golden. Serve immediately.

HAWAIIAN PIZZA

SERVES 4

2 x 400g tins young, green jackfruit in water/brine
250ml BBQ sauce
2 tablespoons tomato purée
1 tablespoon hot sauce
½ teaspoon smoked paprika
1 tablespoon olive oil
salt and pepper
½ red onion, chopped
2-3 cloves garlic, minced
8 sun-dried tomatoes, chopped
260g pineapple chunks
1 vegan pizza base

Pineapple on a pizza is one of those things you either love or you hate. Obviously I love it, hence this recipe. It goes oh so well with the BBQ pulled jackfruit and I can't wait for you to try it if you're in the pineapple on pizzas camp too.

Preheat your oven to 200°C (400°F).

Drain and rinse the jackfruit and use a fork to tear into shreds. Set aside.

In a small bowl combine the BBQ sauce, hot sauce, tomato purée, smoked paprika, and salt and pepper. Mix and then set aside.

Heat 1 tablespoon of olive oil in a frying pan over medium heat for about 1 minute. Add the chopped onion and garlic, and cook for 3-5 minutes until soft.

Add the jackfruit and cook for a further 5 minutes until most of the liquid from jackfruit has gone.

Add the sauce mixture to the jackfruit in the pan, lower the heat to medium-low, cover and leave for about 10-20 minutes, stirring occasionally. Mix in the sun-dried tomatoes and cook for another 2-3 minutes.

Place the pizza dough on a prepared baking tray and spread the jackfruit mixture out evenly. Top with the pineapple chunks and bake for 10-15 minutes in the oven until the crust turns golden. Serve immediately.

TOONA PASTA BAKE

SERVES 4

1 x 400g tins young, green jackfruit in water/brine
1 tablespoon olive oil
2 teaspoons onion powder
2 teaspoons garlic powder
salt and pepper
150g penne pasta
1 x 400g tin coconut milk
1 tablespoon corn flour
170g nutritional yeast
1 x 325g sweet corn (260g drained)
170g dry breadcrumbs

When I was little, my brother and I would often go to our neighbour's house for dinner if my parents were working late. For some reason they always cooked tuna pasta bake, so I have very fond childhood memories of this dish. I was delighted when I was able to closely recreate it for my husband as a vegan version.

Preheat your oven to 180°C (350°F).

Prepare a small baking dish. Drain the jackfruit, rinse well and break up into stringy pieces with a fork.

Heat the olive oil in a frying pan and add the jackfruit, along with 1 teaspoon onion powder, 1 teaspoon garlic powder, and a good seasoning with salt and pepper. Cook until the edges begin to brown and the jackfruit is soft. Set aside.

Next cook the pasta by filling a saucepan with lightly salted water and bring to the boil. Add the pasta and cook for 10 minutes until al dente. Drain and set aside.

Using the same saucepan over a medium heat, add the coconut milk, remaining onion powder, garlic powder, salt, pepper, nutritional yeast and corn flour. Whisk constantly over the heat until the sauce thickens.

Add the sweet corn, jackfruit and pasta to the sauce and mix well. Pour the mixture into the baking tray and spread out evenly. Sprinkle the top with breadcrumbs.

Bake in the oven for 20-30 minutes or until golden brown on top. Serve immediately.

SUSHI ROLLS

MAKES 32 ROLLS
1 x 400g tin young, green jackfruit in water/brine
1 tablespoon tamari
2 ½ teaspoons sriracha
2 tablespoon nutritional yeast
3 tablespoons vegenaise
1 ½ teaspoons sesame oil
4 sheets of nori
700g cooked sushi rice
1 avocado, sliced
ginger and wasabi, to serve

Vegan sushi is refreshingly light and versatile. This jackfruit recipe is one to get you rolling.
Drain the jackfruit and rinse well. Break up the pieces with a fork so they become stringy.
In a saucepan, cover the jackfruit with water. Add in the tamari, 1 teaspoon of sriracha, and nutritional yeast. Put on a medium heat and simmer for 15-20 minutes.
Remove from heat and rinse the jackfruit. Squeeze out any excess liquid in a colander.
In a bowl, mix the jackfruit with the vegenaise, 1½ teaspoons sriracha, and sesame oil. Refrigerate until ready to use.
Making sushi rolls isn't as daunting as you think but if you haven't done it before then I suggest watching a quick YouTube video first.
Place the nori on a sushi mat and spread 3 tablespoons prepared sushi rice on the nori. Place 3 tablespoons of spicy jackfruit and 1/4 of the sliced avocado horizontally, close to the bottom of the nori.
Roll the sushi. Use some water to help the edge of the seaweed stick if needed.
Slice the sushi roll into eight pieces. Serve with pickled ginger and wasabi.

VIETNAMESE ROLLS WITH PEANUT DIP

MAKES 14 ROLLS
FOR THE JACKFRUIT

2 x 400g tins young, green jackfruit in water/brine
100ml hoisin sauce
4 tablespoons tamari
3 tablespoons rice vinegar
3 tablespoons maple syrup
2 tablespoons tomato purée
1 tablespoon sriracha
2 teaspoons corn flour
2 tablespoons sesame oil
5 shallots, diced
2 garlic cloves, minced
1 teaspoon Chinese 5 spice

FOR THE SUMMER ROLLS

14 sheets of rice paper
100g rice vermicelli noodles, cooked and rinsed in cold water
2 medium carrots, peeled and sliced into matchsticks
½ cucumber, sliced into thin sticks
1 head of iceberg lettuce, leaves chopped into 1-inch strips
6 tablespoons coriander, roughly chopped

FOR THE PEANUT DIP

6 tablespoons smooth peanut butter
3½ tablespoons lime juice
3 tablespoons water
2 tablespoons hoisin sauce
2 tablespoons tamari
1-2 teaspoons sriracha

If you're not familiar with these little delicacies then my, you've got a treat in store. They are so light and fresh - a jumble of crunchy raw vegetables, tasty, tender jackfruit, and cool, squidgy noodles, all stuffed snugly into a feather light rice wrapper.

Preheat your oven to 200°C (400°F).

Drain the jackfruit and rinse well. Use a fork to break up the pieces. Set aside.

In a small bowl, whisk together 2 tablespoons hoisin sauce, tamari, rice vinegar, maple syrup, tomato purée, sriracha, until smooth. Whisk in the corn flour until fully incorporated. Set aside. Heat the sesame oil in a large, shallow saucepan over medium heat. Add the chopped shallots and cook for around 5 minutes until the shallots begin to turn translucent. Add the garlic and Chinese 5 spice cook for a couple more minutes.

Add the jackfruit to the pan and cook for 5 minutes, stirring occasionally. Once softened a bit, use two forks to tear the jackfruit into smaller, more shredded pieces. Add the other 2 tablespoons of hoisin sauce and stir until combined. Cook for a couple of minutes.

Meanwhile, prepare a baking tray with baking paper. Spread the jackfruit out into an even layer. Place the tray in the oven and bake for about 25 minutes, turning the pieces halfway through. Once done, remove from the oven and leave to cool for about 10 minutes.

While the jackfruit is baking, prepare the peanut dip. In a medium bowl, whisk together all the sauce ingredients until completely smooth. Chill until ready to use.

To assemble the rolls, fill a wide bowl full of warm water. Dip one of the sheets of rice paper into the water and lay it out on a clean surface. Lay out about 3 tablespoons of the jackfruit mixture into a small strip on the half of the rice paper closest to you. Top with a small handful of the noodles. Lay out several carrot and cucumber sticks next to the noodles, top with a couple strips of lettuce, and then add a sprig of coriander. Fold the edge of rice paper closest to you over the pile. Fold the two side edges towards the centre, and then roll until it is completely sealed. Repeat with the remaining rice paper sheets and ingredients until all are completed. Can be refrigerated for up to 2 days.

SWEET AND STICKY CHINESE JACKFRUIT

SERVES 2

1 x 400g tin young, green jackfruit in water/brine
2 tablespoons rice flour
2 garlic cloves, minced
1 thumb of fresh ginger, peeled and minced
3 tablespoons tamari
3 tablespoons maple syrup
3 tablespoons coconut sugar
1 tablespoon rice vinegar
1 tablespoon corn flour
1½ teaspoons Chinese 5 spice
1 red chilli, deseeded and finely minced
vegetable oil
sesame seeds, to garnish (optional)

This recipe uses the same technique for cooking meat by coating the jackfruit in flour then searing in hot oil for a crispy exterior whilst still tender on the inside. It's great as a starter or easily served with rice and grilled vegetables for a full meal.

Drain and rinse the jackfruit then transfer to a chopping board. Cut into bite sized pieces. Squeeze out as much liquid as possible either with a tea towel or in a colander.

Mince the garlic, ginger and chilli, and then combine in a bowl with the tamari, maple syrup, coconut sugar, vinegar, corn flour, and Chinese 5 spice. Set aside.

Heat a pan over high heat and pour in 2-3 tablespoons of oil.

Whilst the oil is heating in the pan, place the jackfruit in a mixing bowl and sprinkle the rice flour over it and toss. Once it's coated, place in the hot pan one by one. Cook for 2-3 minutes until golden brown on all sides.

Pour in the marinade and lower the heat to medium. Once it starts to bubble, tilt the pan slightly towards you, and spoon the sauce over top the jackfruit .The sauce will start to thicken after a minute or two. Once all the pieces are coated and the sauce has thickened nicely, take off the heat and serve immediately sprinkled with sesame seeds

CRISPY PEKING JACK PANCAKES

SERVES 4

FOR THE JACKFRUIT

2 x 400g tins young, green jackfruit in water/brine
2 tablespoons vegetable oil
2 spring onions, finely chopped
3 cloves garlic, minced
1 thumb-sized piece fresh ginger, minced
1 teaspoon Chinese five spice
2-3 tablespoons tamari
3 tablespoons hoisin sauce
2 teaspoons toasted sesame oil
2 teaspoon rice vinegar
1 teaspoon chilli flakes
pepper, to taste

FOR THE REST

pack of pancakes for crispy duck
hoisin sauce, to serve
1 cucumber, cored and cut into matchsticks
1 spring onion, cut into thin strips lengthwise

For the best flavour with this dish, leave the jackfruit to marinade overnight. It's simply delicious and one that non-meat eaters can't get enough of.

Drain and rinse the jackfruit. Set aside.

Heat up vegetable oil in a large frying pan over a medium heat. Fry the spring onions for 2-3 minutes until softened. Add the minced garlic and ginger and fry until soft and fragrant. Add the Chinese five spice mix for an extra minute, stirring the whole time.

Add the prepared jackfruit along with the tamari, 2 tablespoons hoisin sauce, toasted sesame oil and rice vinegar. Mix everything together in the pan. Squash the jackfruit pieces with your mixing spoon so that the individual fibres break up and soak up more of the sauce. Season with pepper and a pinch of chilli flakes.

Simmer the mixture gently for another 5-10 minutes and then leave to cool. This can be placed in the fridge overnight to intensify the flavour.

When you are ready to make the pancakes, preheat your oven to 200°C (400°F).

Spread the jackfruit pieces on a baking paper-lined baking tray and brush them lightly with an extra tablespoon of hoisin sauce. Bake for 25 minutes, until they look caramelised and have browned around the edges. Remove from the oven and set aside.

Meanwhile, warm up your pancakes in a bamboo steamer or in the microwave.

Smear a bit of hoisin sauce on the inside of each pancake, followed by jackfruit 'duck', cucumber and spring onion matchsticks. Roll up and enjoy with extra hoisin dip on the side if you wish.

STEAMED CHAR SIU BAO BUNS

MAKES 10 BUNS
FOR THE DOUGH
1 teaspoon active dry yeast
175ml warm water
6 tablespoons sugar
700g flour
350g corn flour
2½ teaspoons baking powder
60ml canola oil
cooking oil spray
FOR THE FILLING
1 x 400g tin young, green jackfruit in water/brine
1½ tablespoons sesame oil
2 shallots finely chopped
2½ tablespoons hoisin sauce
1 tablespoon sugar
1 tablespoon tamari
1 teaspoon sriracha
sesame seeds to garnish (optional)

Pillowy and soft meets sweet and tangy. This is an amazing version of this Chinese street food. The dough can also be made up to two months ahead and steamed directly from the freezer in five minutes.

First, make the dough. Combine the yeast, warm water, and ½ teaspoon of sugar in the bowl of an electric mixer fitted with a hook attachment. Mix for around 5 minutes until the yeast is slightly foamy.

Combine the flour, corn flour, remaining 5 tablespoons sugar, and baking powder, stirring with a whisk. Add to the yeast mixture with the canola oil and stir with the dough hook on low for around 3 minutes until everything is fully mixed.

Remove the dough from the bowl and knead gently on a clean work surface for around 5 minutes until smooth. Place in a large bowl coated with cooking spray and cover with a damp cloth. Leave in a warm place for an hour until the dough has doubled in size.

For the filling, heat 1-tablespoon sesame oil in a large frying pan over a medium-high heat. Add the chopped shallot and cook for 1 minute, stirring constantly. Add the drained jackfruit and cook for about 5 minutes until it starts to crisp. Reduce the heat to medium and add the hoisin sauce, sugar, tamari, remaining 1½ teaspoons sesame oil, and sriracha. Cook for a further minute, stirring frequently, until the mixture comes to a simmer. Remove from heat.

Cut a large piece of baking paper into 10 (4x4-inch) squares and set aside. Bring 1 inch of water in your steamer basket to a boil.

Roll the dough into a long log and cut into 10 equal pieces. Flatten each piece into a 4½-inch circle making sure it is thinner around the edges and thicker in the middle. Add 1½ tablespoons of the jackfruit filling and close like a coin purse (4 corners, then remaining 4 corners).

Place each bun on a prepared parchment square and place in the steamer. Steam over high for about 10 minutes until the dough has puffed and is spongy. Serve immediately with a sprinkling of sesame seeds.

SWEET AND SOUR JACKFRUIT

SERVES 6

2 x 400g tins young, green jackfruit in water/brine
500g corn flour
1 teaspoon Chinese five spice
1 teaspoon garlic powder
80ml water
30ml sesame oil
1 red onion, chopped
1 thumb-sized piece fresh ginger, minced
1 green bell pepper, chopped
1 x 400g tin pineapple
4 tablespoons rice vinegar
3 tablespoons ketchup
200g brown sugar
1 spring onion, sliced (optional)

Try this speedy sweet and sour recipe for a Friday night 'fakeaway' or to celebrate Chinese New Year.

In a small bowl, mix the corn flour, Chinese five spice, garlic powder and water. Mix together until it forms a thick-ish creamy consistency.

Drain and rinse the jackfruit. Stir in the jackfruit pieces into the corn flour mix until well coated. Pour the coated jackfruit mix into a frying pan and cook over a medium-high heat for 5 minutes until it starts to crisp at the edges. Transfer to a bowl and set aside.

In the same pan as before, add the sesame oil, chopped red onion, ginger, green bell pepper. Cook for 5-8 minutes until softened. Then add the pineapple juice, rice vinegar, ketchup and sugar, and stir well.

Add the prepared jackfruit and pineapple chunks to the pan. Stir and simmer for 10 minutes until it makes a delicious sticky sauce.

Serve immediately with boiled rice and sliced spring onions on top.

BUTTER CHICK'N

SERVES 2

1 x 400g tin young, green jackfruit in water/brine
1 x 400ml tin coconut milk
1 x 400g tin chopped tomatoes
1 tablespoon vegetable oil
1 large onion, sliced
3 garlic cloves, minced
1 thumb-sized piece fresh ginger, minced
1 tablespoon garam masala
1½ teaspoons ground coriander
1 teaspoon cumin
½ teaspoon chilli flakes
¼ teaspoon cinnamon
1 tablespoon agave syrup
fresh coriander, to garnish

The same creamy, flavourful taste as the original but without the meat and dairy. This can also be made in the slow cooker for added depth of flavour.

Heat the vegetable oil in a medium sized pan over a medium heat. Add the chopped onions and cook for 5-8 minutes until they start to brown, stirring frequently.

Add the minced garlic and ginger to the pan. Stir in the garam masala, ground coriander, cumin, chilli flakes, and cinnamon. Cook for 1-2 minutes.

Meanwhile, drain and rinse the jackfruit then add to the pan with the spices. Cook for a further 3 minutes until the jackfruit is fully coated in the spices.

Pour in the coconut milk, crushed tomatoes, and agave syrup. Stir well and bring to boil, then reduce heat to medium-low and let simmer for 30-35 minute until the sauce has reduced and thickened. If you would like a runnier sauce, just add a splash of water. You can also break up the jackfruit pieces with the back of your spoon if you prefer a shredded effect rather than chunks.

Serve topped with fresh coriander and with fluffy basmati rice.

VEGAN MADRAS

SERVES 2

2 x 400g tins young, green jackfruit in water/brine
4 tablespoons madras curry paste
1 onion, diced
5 garlic cloves, minced
200ml coconut milk
1 x 400g tin chopped tomatoes
vegetable oil
fresh coriander, to garnish

If you like more of a kick in your curry, spicy madras is the way to go. You won't miss meat in this tasty vegan version made with chunks of jackfruit.

Heat the vegetable oil in a medium pan over a medium heat. Add the chopped onions and garlic and cook for 5-8 minutes until soft, stirring frequently.

Drain and rinse the jackfruit. Add the pieces to the pan along with the madras curry paste and cook for 5 minutes. Use the back of your spoon to press against the jackfruit pieces so the fibres separate and absorb more of the paste.

Next, add the chopped tomatoes and coconut milk. Simmer for 30-35 minutes until the jackfruit is tender and the sauce has reduced and thickened.

Serve topped with fresh coriander and fluffy basmati rice.

SRI-LANKAN COCONUT CURRY

SERVES 4

2 x 400g tins young, green jackfruit in water/brine
1 x 400g tin coconut milk
1 red onion, chopped
2 garlic cloves, minced
1 red chilli, finely chopped and seeded
2 tablespoons vegetable oil
1 teaspoon curry powder
½ teaspoon cumin
½ teaspoon ground coriander
¼ teaspoon black pepper
½ teaspoon chilli powder
¾ teaspoon turmeric
½ teaspoon cinnamon
2 bay leaves
120ml water
2 tablespoons lime juice
1 tablespoon agave syrup
pinch of salt
fresh coriander chopped, for garnish

This curry is a real crowd-pleaser. I've made it so many times for dinner parties and it goes down a treat with vegans and meat eaters alike. Double the quantity and freeze for a quick mid-meal meal.

Heat the vegetable oil in a medium pan over a medium heat. Add the chopped onion and fry for 5 minutes until soft, stirring constantly.

Drain and rinse the jackfruit. Tip in to the pan.

Add the garlic, chilli, curry powder, ground cumin, coriander, black pepper, chilli powder, turmeric, and cinnamon. Fry for 2-3 minutes until fragrant and the jackfruit pieces are fully coated.

Add the lime juice, agave syrup and a pinch of salt. Mix well. Fry for 5 minutes, stirring often. Next, add the coconut milk and the bay leaves and reduce the heat to low. Simmer partially covered for 30 minutes until the jackfruit pieces have softened and the sauce has thickened. While cooking, gradually stir in water, if desired, for a thinner curry. Feel free to add any additional vegetables such as bell peppers or runner beans at this point.

Remove bay leaves before serving.

Garnish with fresh coriander and serve with fluffy basmati rice.

BANGLADESHI BIRYANI

SERVES 4

FOR THE MARINADE
1 x 400g tin young, green jackfruit in water/brine
65ml coconut yoghurt
¼ teaspoon chilli powder
½ teaspoon garam masala
20g minced ginger
1 clove garlic, minced
½ tablespoon olive oil

FOR THE RICE
500g white basmati rice
8 green cardamom pods
6 cloves
3 bay leaves
1 teaspoon cumin seeds
pinch of salt

FOR THE BIRYANI
¼ tsp. chilli
200ml coconut yoghurt
1 teaspoon garam masala
2 tablespoons fresh coriander
2 tablespoons fresh mint
1 teaspoon turmeric
1 teaspoon lemon juice
1 onion, diced and cooked

TO TOP
2 tablespoons fresh coriander
2 teaspoons garam masala

Biryani was the first ever jackfruit dish I tried. It was in a restaurant in London with my vegetarian friend. We were intrigued so we ordered it to share. When it came, it tasted so much like meat so I called the waiter over thinking there was a mistake, only to discover this was how convincing the jackfruit was! And so began my love affair with this fruit that ultimately led to this cookbook.

Drain and rinse the jackfruit. Mix together all the ingredients for the marinade. Coat the jackfruit and leave covered with cling film in the fridge for at least 4 hours or ideally overnight.

For the rice, fill a large pot with water. Add all the spices for the rice and then bring the water to a boil.

When the water is boiling, add the rice and stir well. Cook the rice on a medium to high heat for 5 minutes. Take the pan off the heat.

Quickly remove any big pieces of spice floating on top of the water with a sieve.

Strain the rice with a colander and check for any leftover spices and remove them with the help of a fork. Leave the cumin seeds in the rice though.

Transfer the marinated jackfruit from the fridge to a big saucepan. Add in all the ingredients for the biryani, mix well and spread evenly on the bottom of the pan.

Mix the cooked rice with the jackfruit mixture, and then add the fresh coriander and garam masala. Stir and add 100ml water to the dish.

Cover the pot and cook on a medium heat for 10 minutes, then 15 minutes on low heat, stirring occasionally.

Check the rice is fully cooked and add more water if needed and return to heat. When ready, serve immediately with fresh coriander on top.

NANKA RENDANG

SERVES 4
FOR THE MARINADE
2 x 400g tins young, green jackfruit in water/brine
1 x 400g tin chickpeas
2 x 400ml tins coconut milk
2 onions, roughly chopped
4 garlic cloves, chopped
1 thumb-sized piece fresh ginger, minced
3 red chillies, seeded and chopped
1cm piece galangal, roughly chopped
½ teaspoon turmeric
1 bay leaf
1 stalk lemongrass, outer layer removed
1 teaspoon salt

This dish is inspired from our trip to Borneo where fresh jackfruit can be found. Rendang is a typical Indonesian dish; it's so aromatic and packed with flavour.

Place the onion, garlic, ginger, chillies and galangal into a food processor with about 50ml of the coconut milk and process until smooth.

Pour the mixture in to a large saucepan along with the rest of the coconut milk, turmeric, bay leaf, lemongrass, and salt. Drain and rinse the jackfruit. Add to the pan and bring to a boil. Lower the heat to medium-low and leave to simmer uncovered for about 90 minutes, stirring occasionally. After 60 minutes the sauce will become very thick and will require more frequent stirring, scraping the bottom so the jackfruit absorbs it. Continue until all the sauce has been absorbed by the jackfruit.

Add the chickpeas and cook for a further 20 minutes. There should be no liquid remaining. Remove the lemongrass and bay leaf before serving with steamed basmati rice.

GREEN THAI CURRY

SERVES 4

1 x 400g tin young, green jackfruit in water/brine
1 x 400ml tin coconut milk
2 tablespoons of Thai green curry paste
1 onion, chopped
2 garlic cloves, minced
thumb of ginger, minced
2 green chillies, seeded and finely chopped
1 tablespoon coconut oil
2 green bell peppers, sliced
10-12 sugar snap peas, sliced
2 pak choi
½ bunch of fresh coriander

This dish is so easy to throw together for a tasty mid-week meal. Make sure to check the Thai curry paste is vegan (i.e. no fish sauce). Get creative and mix up the vegetables too with alternatives such as baby sweetcorn, green beans, and aubergine.

In a large pan, heat a tablespoon of coconut oil over a medium heat. When melted, add the chopped onion, garlic and chilli. Cook for 3-5 minutes until fragrant.

Drain and rinse the jackfruit then add to the pan along with the ginger. Cook for 8-10 minutes, ensuring the jackfruit pieces are full coated in the spices.

Add Thai green curry paste, green bell peppers, sugar snap peas, and pak choi. When the leaves of the pack choi have wilted down, add in the coconut milk.

Reduce to a simmer and leave for 15 minutes, stirring occasionally.

When finished, add the fresh coriander on top. Serve with steamed rice.

JAMAICAN JERK JACKFRUIT

SERVES 4

1 x 400g tin young, green jackfruit in water/brine
400g tin of kidney beans
200ml coconut milk
1 onion, chopped
2 garlic cloves, minced
1 red chilli, seeded and finely chopped
2 tomatoes, chopped
2 teaspoons Jamaican jerk seasoning
1 tablespoon olive oil
50g baby leaf spinach
salt and pepper
150g white rice
fresh parsley, to garnish (optional)

This is an absolute powerhouse of a vegan dish. It's packed with flavour and very nutritious with the kidney beans upping the protein.

Pour a tablespoon of olive oil into a large pan over a medium heat. Add the chopped onions and a good pinch of salt and pepper. Fry for 4-5 minutes, stirring occasionally, until softened. Stir in the garlic, chilli and 2 teaspoons Jamaican jerk seasoning and continue to fry for a further 2 minutes.

Drain and rinse the jackfruit then add to the pan. Stir for 2-3 minutes until fully coated in the spices.

Pour in the coconut milk and chopped tomatoes Combine well and bring to the boil, then reduce the heat to simmer for 20-25 minutes. During the cooking time, use your spoon every now and then to break up the jackfruit chunks so they absorb more flavour.

Drain and rinse the kidney beans. Add them to the pan halfway through cooking and mix in. After you've added the kidney beans, bring a small pan of water to boil. When boiling, add the rice and cook for 10 minutes.

Meanwhile, stir the spinach into the jackfruit mix until it has wilted.

Serve the jackfruit with the rice and a sprinkling of fresh parsley on top.

Drain the rice and serve with a large spoonful of the jackfruit mix.

JERK BLACK BEAN AND MANGO WRAP

MAKES 3-4 WRAPS

JERK JACKFRUIT
1 x 400g tin young, green jackfruit in water/brine
2 teaspoons olive oil
1 teaspoon dried thyme
1 teaspoon dried parsley
1 teaspoon paprika
½ teaspoon cayenne
¼ teaspoon cinnamon
¼ teaspoon nutmeg
1 teaspoon lime juice
450ml water
½ teaspoon sugar
salt and pepper

BLACK BEANS
1 teaspoon olive oil
1 onion, chopped
2 cloves garlic, minced
1 x 400g tin black beans
1 teaspoon dried thyme
1 teaspoon dried parsley
½ teaspoon cayenne
1 teaspoon lime juice
50 ml water

OTHER FILLINGS
chopped mango
fresh coriander
large tortilla wraps

This light, healthy wrap is a deliciously exotic way to enjoy a variation on the burrito. It can be gluten free too if you choose gluten-free wraps.

Drain and rinse the jackfruit. Chop in to small pieces and break up the fibres with a fork. Put in a container with the thyme, parsley, cayenne, cinnamon, nutmeg, and lime juice. Leave in the fridge to marinade for 1 hour minimum or overnight for maximum flavour.

Heat 2 teaspoons olive oil in a frying pan over medium heat. Add the marinated jackfruit and cook for 2-3 minutes until fragrant.

Add the water and sugar and cook for 25 to 30 minutes until the water has evaporated and the mixture is dry. Taste and adjust with more seasoning if you want.

While the jackfruit is cooking, prepare the black beans. Heat 1 teaspoon olive oil in a separate frying pan over a medium heat. Add the chopped onions and garlic and cook for 3-5 minutes until golden. Add the black beans, thyme, parsley, cayenne, lime juice and water to the pan. Simmer for 10 minutes, stirring occasionally.

When the black beans and jackfruit are ready, layer a spoonful of each in the centre of a large tortilla wrap. Top with fresh coriander and mango. Fold into a burrito and serve immediately.

NOT-JUST-MUSHROOM STROGANOFF

SERVES 6

1 x 400g tin young, green jackfruit in water/brine
2 tablespoons olive oil
1 onion, diced
100g dried mushrooms
200g chestnut mushrooms
4-5 garlic cloves, minced
250ml red wine
75g raw cashews
250ml vegetable stock
½ teaspoon dried thyme
350ml mushroom gravy
salt and pepper
fresh parsley

This sauce is so scrumptious and creamy. The jackfruit does a brilliant job of replacing beef to bring out all the flavours in this one pot. It can also be easily made in a slow cooker.

In a large pan, heat the olive oil over a medium heat. Add the chopped onion and garlic and cook for 5-8 minutes until soft.

Next, add the chestnut and dried mushrooms. Cover and cook for 10 minutes.

Add the red wine, stir in, and cook for a further 5 minutes.

Rinse and drain the jackfruit, and then add to the pan.

Meanwhile, blend the cashews with the vegetable stock with a hand blender. Add to the pan along with the mushroom gravy, thyme, and a pinch of salt and pepper. Stir and cover. Cook on medium-low for 20-25 minutes, stirring occasionally and using the back of your spoon to gently break up the jackfruit.

Serve immediately topped with fresh parsley and with either pasta, crusty bread, or rice.

VEGAN GYROS

MAKES 6 GYROS
FOR THE JACKFRUIT
2 x 400g tins young, green jackfruit in water/brine
4 tablespoons olive oil
1 red onion, finely diced
4 garlic cloves, minced
¼ teaspoon ground cloves
¼ teaspoon ground cinnamon
½ teaspoon ground cumin
2 teaspoons dry oregano
½ teaspoon chilli power
2 tablespoons tomato puree
4 tablespoons tamari
2 tablespoons maple syrup
salt and pepper
2 teaspoons apple cider vinegar
OTHER INGREDIENTS
½ cucumber, sliced
100g cherry tomatoes, quartered
vegan tzatziki
6 large Greek pitta breads
6 Romaine lettuce leaves, shredded
1 small red onion, finely sliced
olive oil

Gyros are quintessentially a meat-lover's choice, but it turns out that the mighty jackfruit has made it totally possible for vegans too. For the best flavour, marinade the jackfruit a day ahead. Heat 2 tablespoons of olive oil in a medium pan. Fry the diced red onion for 5 minutes until soft and translucent. Add the minced garlic and fry for a further 2 minutes until fragrant.

Add most of the spices: cloves, cinnamon, cumin, and oregano. Cook for a further minute or so, stirring constantly. Mix in the tomato puree.

Drain both jackfruit tins and rinse thoroughly. Add to the pan along with the tamari, maple syrup and apple cider vinegar. Mix everything together. Squash the jackfruit pieces with your mixing spoon or a fork so that the individual fibres separate.

Simmer the mixture gently for another 10-15 minutes so the sauce thickens and then allow it to cool down. Place in the fridge overnight to intensify the flavour.

When you are ready to prepare your gyros, preheat the oven to 200°C (400°F). Spread the jackfruit pieces in a single layer on a lined baking tray and cook for about 20-25 minutes. The jackfruit should start to caramelise and brown around the edges. If you would like it to be crispier at this point, transfer to a frying pan and cook on a high heat for 3-5 minutes until the edges begin to crisp up. Set aside.

Warm the pitta breads up in the oven for 2-3 minutes.

Remove the pittas and place on a work surface. Make an insert along the top to cut open lengthways. Fill with lettuce, cucumber, tomato, onion, and baked jackfruit. Serve with a generous dollop of tzatziki.

JACKFRUIT 'LAMB' TAGINE

SERVES 8

1 x 400g tin young, green jackfruit in water/brine
1 x 400g tin chickpeas
1 large onion, thinly sliced
1 tablespoon olive oil
1 thumb sized piece fresh ginger, thinly sliced
1 garlic clove, minced
½ teaspoon turmeric
½ teaspoon cayenne pepper
½ teaspoon cinnamon
1 teaspoon cumin powder
1 teaspoon paprika
1 tablespoon tomato puree
1 teaspoon ras el hanout
1 litre vegetable stock
170g dried apricots
100g golden raisins
2 tablespoons chopped parsley
salt and pepper

This is the speedier version for this recipe but it also works brilliantly in a slow cooker. Make sure to marinade the jackfruit first though so it fully soaks up the flavours.

Mix the garlic, ginger, turmeric, paprika, salt and cumin powder. Drain and rinse the jackfruit, then mix the pieces in the spices and set aside.

Heat the olive oil in a large saucepan. Add the chopped onions and cook on a medium heat for 5 minutes until softened. Add a pinch of salt to sweeten the onions.

Stir in the tomato puree and cook for a further 2-3 minutes.

Add the marinated jackfruit pieces. Cook on a medium-high heat for 10 minutes, stirring frequently.

Add the vegetable stock. There should be enough to almost cover the jackfruit. Now add the drained chickpeas, apricots, raisins, cayenne pepper, cinnamon, and ras el hanout. Stir well, cover and cook for 25-30 minutes.

Check whilst cooking if the sauce looks too dry and the remaining stock or water if necessary. Garnish with parsley, and serve with fluffy couscous.

NANA'S HOT POT

SERVES 6

1 x 400g tin young, green jackfruit in water/brine
400g potatoes, diced into 1 inch cubes
½ onion, chopped
2 tablespoons olive oil
5 garlic cloves, minced
1 large carrot, thickly sliced
1 ½ litres vegetable stock
2 teaspoons chilli powder
3-4 teaspoons smoked paprika
3 bay leaves
2 teaspoons dried oregano
10 sprigs thyme
handful fresh parsley, chopped
salt and pepper

This hearty delicious stew from my hometown near Manchester gives me all the feels. I was overjoyed when jackfruit was able to replace the texture of the lamb normally used for this dish.

Pour the olive oil into a medium casserole dish on a medium heat. Add the chopped onion. Cook for about 5 minutes until soft and translucent.

Stir in the chopped carrot and the garlic and stir for another 1-2 minutes until fragrant.

Drain and rinse the jackfruit, and then add the pieces to the dish. Stir in the chilli powder, smoked paprika, oregano, thyme and bay leaves. Stir well so the jackfruit is evenly coated and cook for 3-5 minutes until soft.

Pour in the vegetable stock and bring down to a simmer. Cover with a lid and cook for 40 minutes.

At this point you can use a fork or the back of your spoon to help break up the jackfruit pieces. Add the potatoes and cook for another 15 minutes or until the potatoes are tender. Taste and adjust seasonings with more salt and/or pepper if needed.

Remove from heat and discard the bay leaves and thyme sprigs. Stir in most of the parsley, reserving some for garnish. Serve immediately and enjoy.

CHICK'N AND MUSHROOM PIE

SERVES 4
FOR THE FILLING
1 x 400g tin young, green jackfruit in water/brine
300ml unsweetened almond milk
½ onion, diced
2 garlic cloves, minced
2 bay leaves
2 sprigs of rosemary
1 tablespoon olive oil
150g potatoes, diced into small chunks
150g carrots, cut into chunks
200g frozen peas
FOR THE ROUX
40g plain flour
40g vegan butter
300ml unsweetened almond milk
50g puff pastry
1 teaspoon vegan butter, melted

This vegan 'chicken' and mushroom pie will leave you feeling warm and cosy on the inside and smiling on the outside. Enjoy!

Heat the olive oil in a large pan on a medium heat and add the onion. Fry for 5 minutes until softened.

Drain and rinse the jackfruit, and then add to the pan along with the minced garlic, bay leaves, rosemary, and almond milk. Reduce the heat and simmer for 25 minutes until the jackfruit has softened. Use a fork or a potato masher to shred the jackfruit.

Add the chopped carrots, potatoes and peas. Turn the heat back up to medium and simmer for another 15-20 minutes until all the vegetables have softened.

Remove the pan from the heat. Using a slotted spoon, discard the bay leaves and rosemary. Then scoop out the jackfruit and vegetables into a large bowl. Strain the remaining mixture through a sieve into a large jug.

Preheat the oven to 200°C (400°F).

Using the same pan, wipe it clean, and heat a small knob of vegan butter. Once it's all melted, whisk together with the flour until it forms a paste. Cook for 2 minutes.

Pour in half (150ml) almond milk and bring to boil. After 2 minutes of boiling, reduce the heat to low and then whisk until the roux starts to thicken.

Once all the lumps are gone, add the other half of the almond milk. Whisk again until smooth. Remove from the heat and stir in the vegetables.

Pour the mixture into a deep casserole dish. Roll out the puff pastry on a surface so it's large enough to cover the top of the dish. Lay over the top of the dish and press down the sides with your fingers to secure.

Brush the top of the pastry with a bit of melted butter. Cut two slits in the middle of the pastry. Bake for 20 minutes until the pastry is golden brown. Serve immediately.

GUINESSS IRISH STEW

SERVES 8

1 x 400g tin young, green jackfruit in water/brine
1 x 440ml can of Guinness
3 teaspoons olive oil
1 bay leaf
5 garlic cloves, minced
1 onion, finely chopped
5 medium potatoes, chopped
4 large carrots, diced
4 large celery stalks, diced
800ml vegetable stock
3 tablespoons tomato puree
1 sprig fresh rosemary
salt and pepper
4 tablespoons corn flour

A dish you simply must make to celebrate St Patricks' day with friends and family. It can easily be made in advanced and heated through in the oven.

Heat a teaspoon of olive oil in large frying pan over a medium heat. Add the bay leaf and minced garlic. Simmer for 1-2 minutes until fragrant. Remove the bay leaf and discard.

Add the chopped onion and cook for 5 minutes until translucent, stirring often.

Drain and rinse the jackfruit, and then add to the pan with a pinch of salt and pepper. Cook for 5 minutes until softened. Use a fork or the back of your spoon to help break up the pieces.

Meanwhile, add the vegetable stock to a large saucepan over a high heat. Add the chopped potatoes and bring to a boil. Reduce the heat to medium and transfer the jackfruit mix.

Add in the chopped celery, carrots, tomato puree, and a sprig of rosemary. Cook over a medium heat for a further 5 minutes. Finally, add the Guinness, stir and reduce heat to low. Leave to simmer partially covered for 1-2 hours (this can also be done for longer in a slow cooker).

Mix 4 tablespoons corn flour with a tablespoon of water in a small bowl so it makes a paste. Transfer this paste to the saucepan, stirring constantly. Bring to a boil whilst continuing to stir and the sauce thickens.

Serve immediately with some warm, crusty bread.

JACKFRUIT AND STOUT COTTAGE PIE

SERVES 4

1 x 400g tin young, green jackfruit in water/brine
250ml dark stout
170g plain flour
1 large carrot, diced
100g mushrooms, sliced
1 stalk of celery, diced
1 medium onion, chopped
1 garlic clove, chopped
1 tablespoon tomato puree
1 large tomato, chopped
1 tablespoon nutritional yeast
3 sprigs of thyme – leaves only
1 tablespoon tamari
1 teaspoon dried parsley
¼ teaspoon marjoram
1 tablespoon olive oil
1 teaspoon paprika
150ml water
500g red skinned potatoes – scrubbed
60ml unsweetened almond milk
25g vegan butter
nutritional yeast (optional)
salt and pepper, to taste

This scrumptious vegan pie is hearty and comforting. Add parsnips to the mash to increase your veg intake if you want. Serve with garden peas.

Drain and rinse the jackfruit. Transfer to a bowl and pour over the stout. Leave to marinade for at least one hour (the longer you leave it, the more intense the flavour).

When you are ready to cook, drain the stout from the jackfruit and reserve in a jug. Mix the flour in with the jackfruit, coating well.

Heat the oil in a large frying pan over a medium heat. Cook the jackfruit for about 5 minutes until browned, stirring frequently. Remove from the pan and set aside in a dish.

In the same pan, add the chopped onions, celery, carrot and garlic and cook for 2-3 minutes until slightly softened. Then add the mushrooms, tomato puree, chopped tomato, nutritional yeast, thyme, tamari, parsley, marjoram, paprika, and 150ml water. Bring to a simmer and then finally add the reserved stout and the jackfruit. Mix well, then cover and simmer for about 30 minutes over a low heat, stirring often.

Preheat your oven to 180°C (350°F).

Spoon the mixture into an ovenproof dish.

Next, prepare the potato topping. Chop the potatoes into large chunks, and then add to a pan of lightly salted water. Bring to a boil and cook for 15 minutes until tender. Drain and add the almond milk and vegan butter. Mash until creamy. Season to taste.

Spoon the mashed potato over the top of the base mixture and glide a fork across the surface. Sprinkle with some nutritional yeast for a hint of 'cheesy' flavour.

Bake for 40-45 minutes until the top is crisp and gold. Serve immediately with a side of garden peas.

STUFFED PEPPERS

SERVES 4

1 x 400g tin young, green jackfruit in water/brine
4 x bean burgers
4 bell peppers
1 tablespoon olive oil
1 teaspoon salt
128g grated vegan cheese
½ teaspoon ground cumin
½ teaspoon paprika
½ oregano
1 avocado, sliced
fresh coriander, chopped

Colourful, packed with flavour, and perfect for a quick lunch or dinner. The secret to the speediness of these stuffed peppers is buying ready-made bean burgers to mix together with the jackfruit. Top with melted vegan cheese and some avocado and you've got a wholesome plant-based plate.

Preheat oven to 180°C (350°F).

Cut off the tops of the peppers but don't throw them away. Remove the seeds and membranes and discard. Brush the peppers with some olive oil and sprinkle with salt.

Line a baking tray, then cook the peppers and bean burgers in the oven under a closed grill. This should take 10 minutes until they are charred on both sides. Flip the burgers halfway through. Set aside.

Meanwhile, prepare the jackfruit. Drain and rinse well, then chop up the pieces on a chopping board. Transfer to a frying pan along with the cumin, paprika, and oregano. Cook for 5-8 minutes until soft. Use a fork or your spoon to help break up the pieces.

Crumble the bean burgers into a bowl. Evenly fill the peppers with the jackfruit and bean burger mix. Sprinkle with cheese. Pop under the grill for a minute if the cheese doesn't melt straight away. Serve topped with avocado and fresh coriander.

LOADED NACHOS

SERVES 4-6

2 x 400g tins young, green jackfruit in water/brine
200g tortilla chips (suitable for vegans)
170ml BBQ sauce
150g grated vegan cheese
½ red onion, diced
10 cherry tomatoes, halved
fresh coriander, chopped
handful of jalapeños
guacamole
vegan sour cream (optional)

How about these for your next get together with friends? Or to appease your weeknight craving for nachos? (been there, often).

Preheat oven to 180°C (350°F).

Drain and rinse the jackfruit. Cut out the hard core and chop it into small pieces (don't throw it away!).

Add the jackfruit, BBQ sauce, and 50ml water into a hot frying pan and simmer for 20 minutes until the jackfruit is soft and the sauce has thickened. Squash the jackfruit in the pan with a fork or a spoon to help further shred the pieces.

Lay out half of the nachos out on a baking tray. Scoop on half of the jackfruit mix, along with some vegan cheese, red onion, and cherry tomatoes. Layer the remaining nachos on top, with the rest of the jackfruit, cheese, onion, and tomatoes. Bake for 15 minutes in the preheated oven. Remove the nachos from the oven and top with jalapenos, coriander, guacamole and sour cream. Serve and enjoy.

JACK AND THE BLACK BEANS ENCHILADAS

SERVES 4

1 x 400g tin young, green jackfruit in water/brine
1 x 400g tin black beans
1 x 215g jar of jalapenos
1 x 500g carton passata/tomato sauce
2 garlic cloves, minced
½ onion, diced
1 teaspoon cumin
1 teaspoon smoked paprika
1 teaspoon chilli powder
salt and pepper
2 tablespoons olive oil
2 handfuls of baby spinach
8 tortillas
340g grated vegan cheese
fresh coriander, chopped
sliced avocado (optional)

Truly delicious and packed with protein, these vegan enchiladas are perfect for the whole family.
Drain and rinse the jackfruit. Pull the pieces apart with a fork so it resembles pulled pork. Set aside.
Preheat the oven to 200°C (400°F).
Pour 2 tablespoons of olive oil in a large frying pan over and a medium heat. Add the chopped onion and garlic and cook for 2-3 minutes until soft and fragrant.
Add the jackfruit pieces along with the cumin, chilli powder, and smoked paprika. Cook for 5 minutes until most of the moisture from the jackfruit has evaporated.
Drain the black beans, and then add these to the pan along with the jalapenos. Cook for another 2-3 minutes, using your spoon to mash up some of the beans against the edge of the pan.
Stir in the baby spinach and cook until just wilted for 1 minute. Remove from heat.
In a medium baking dish, pour in half of the tomato sauce. Take the tortillas and place a large dollop of the jackfruit mix in the centre of each tortilla. Roll up the tortillas and place them seam-side down in the dish. Pour the other half of the tomato sauce on top to cover the tortillas. Sprinkle with vegan cheese.
Bake for 25-30 minutes. Serve the enchiladas warm with fresh coriander and sliced avocado.

SLOW-COOKER STUFFED SWEET POTATOES

SERVES 4

2 x 400g tins young, green jackfruit in water/brine
4 large sweet potatoes
1 tablespoon brown sugar
1 teaspoon dried oregano
1 teaspoon cumin
½ teaspoon smoked paprika
½ teaspoon chilli powder
250ml vegan BBQ sauce
fresh coriander, to garnish

This recipe is so simple to make as the slow cooker does all the work. It's packed with flavour and I simply love the contrast of the smoky meatiness of the jackfruit with the smooth sweet potato.

Drain and rinse the jackfruit. Tip the jackfruit pieces in to a large mixing bowl and add in the sugar, oregano, cumin, paprika, and chilli powder. Stir so that the jackfruit is coated. Transfer to the slow cooker, pour over the BBQ sauce and give it another stir.

Cook on low for 5-6 hours.

After 5 hours, shred the jackfruit with a fork. Cook for an additional hour.

Meanwhile, preheat the oven to 180°C (350°F). Prick the sweet potatoes with a fork and wrap them in tin foil. Place on a baking tray and cook for 45 minutes.

Serve the cooked jackfruit over the baked sweet potatoes and serve with a crispy side salad.

TIP: I love to make extra of the slow-cooked jackfruit as it's so versatile for many of the other recipes in this book too. It can be kept in the fridge for 2-3 days or in the freeze for 1 month. Defrost overnight before cooking and add a splash of water to the pan so that it doesn't dry out.

SWEET CHILLI SPRING ROLLS

SERVES 4

1 x 400g tin young, green jackfruit in water/brine
18-20 square mini spring roll wrappers
1 tablespoon sesame oil
170g dried mushrooms
2 garlic cloves, minced
1 thumb-sized piece of ginger, peeled and chopped
2 spring onions, finely sliced
1 pak choi
1 medium carrot, cut into matchstick pieces
350g beansprouts
1 teaspoon Chinese 5 spice
3 tablespoon tamari
1 tablespoon lime juice
1 tablespoon coriander, finely chopped
2 tablespoons corn flour
1 tablespoon vegetable oil
sweet chilli sauce (to serve)

Meaty, sweet and savoury pulled jackfruit meets crunchy and delicious in these spring rolls that will have you wishing you'd made more!

Soak the dried mushrooms in a small bowl of boiling water.

Pre-heat the oven to 180°C (350°F) and line a baking tray with greaseproof paper.

Drain and rinse the jackfruit, cut into small pieces and set aside.

Heat a tablespoon of sesame oil in a frying pan over a medium heat. Add the minced garlic, ginger, spring onions, and Chinese 5 spice. Cook for 2-3 minutes until fragrant, and then add the jackfruit pieces. Stir to make sure the jackfruit pieces are well coated and use a fork or the back of your spoon to push down the pieces and break up the fibres.

Next, add the leaves from the pak choi, the carrot matchstick pieces and the beansprouts. Cook on a medium heat for 10 minutes, stirring often.

Meanwhile, drain and chop the dried mushrooms and add along with the tamari, lime juice, coriander and corn flour. Mix well and cook for 5 more minutes, stirring constantly. Remove from heat.

Place a spring roll wrap on a chopping board with one of the corners facing towards you. Place 1 tablespoon of the jackfruit mixture across the left and right corners in an oblong, sausage shape. Fold the corner that is pointing towards you over the mixture. Fold in the two sides and then push away from you to roll up fully. Use a splash of water on the edge of the wrapper to secure if needed.

Place each spring roll on a lined baking tray and brush with vegetable oil. Bake for 25 minutes, until golden and crispy.

Serve immediately with sweet chilli sauce.

SMOKY PULLED-NOT-PORK TACOS

SERVES 4

FOR THE FILLING

2 x 400g tins young, green jackfruit in water/brine
2 tablespoons coconut oil
½ onion, thinly sliced
4 garlic cloves, minced
1 tablespoon smoked paprika
1 tablespoon ground cumin
1 tablespoon chilli powder
2-3 tablespoons maple syrup
1-2 red or green chillies, chopped
3 teaspoons hot habanero sauce
3 tablespoons lime juice

FOR SERVING

8 tacos
1 x 400g tin refried pinto or black beans
chopped avocado
fresh coriander
lime wedges
salsa
hot habanero sauce

Tacos have become one of the most popular recipes to make with jackfruit, and there's a reason for it – they're so tasty! The meatiness of the jackfruit perfectly marries with the crunchiness of the tacos. Go wild with the heat you handle. Any leftover jackfruit can be stored in the fridge for 4-5 days or frozen and defrosted overnight before cooking.

Rinse and drain the jackfruit. Transfer to a chopping board and cut into small pieces. Pull the pieces apart with either a fork or your fingers to resemble pulled pork.

Heat a large frying pan over medium heat with a tablespoon of coconut oil. Once hot, add in the chopped onion, garlic, and chillies. Cook for 4-5 minutes until fragrant and the onions have softened.

Add the jackfruit to the pan along with the paprika, cumin, chilli powder, maple syrup and lime juice. Coat the jackfruit in the spices and cook for 3-5 minutes. Add in 50ml of water then reduce the heat and cover for 20 minutes, stirring occasionally.

As your jackfruit is cooking and begins to soften, you can continue to break up the pieces with a fork or a spoon to give it more of a 'stringy' pulled meat effect.

Taste and adjust the flavour as needed – add some habanero sauce for spiciness, more paprika for smokiness, or lime juice for acidity. Cook for a further 2-3 minutes then remove from heat. Serve up in tacos with toppings of your choice – I love refried beans, salsa and extra habanero sauce!

MEATLESS TIKKA MASALA

SERVES 4

1 x 400g tin young, green jackfruit in water/brine
1 x 400g tin chopped tomatoes
1 x 400g tin coconut milk
1 medium onion, chopped
6-8 garlic cloves, finely chopped
1 teaspoon cumin seeds
1 teaspoon chilli powder
1 teaspoon ground coriander
1 teaspoon garam masala
½ teaspoon cinnamon
vegetable oil
fresh coriander to garnish
coconut yoghurt (optional)

Healthy Indian food at home that's better than a takeaway. It's creamy, spicy, and meaty despite being completely plant-based! Enjoy with fluffy basmati rice and vegan parathas.

Preheat the oven to 200°C (400°F).

Rinse and drain the jackfruit, then cut into smaller, bite-sizes.

Mix the chilli powder, coriander, cinnamon and garam masala in a large bowl. Tip in the jackfruit pieces in and coat on all sides.

Spread the seasoned jackfruit out on a lightly greased baking sheet and bake for 20 minutes.

Meanwhile, pour 1 tablespoon of vegetable oil in a large saucepan on a medium heat. Add the cumin seeds for 1-2 minutes until they begin to crack. Add the chopped onion and garlic and cook for 3-5 minutes until soft.

Add the jackfruit from the oven into the pan and stir for 1-2 minutes. Next, add in the chopped tomatoes and coconut milk. Mix well, then cover and reduce the heat to simmer. Leave to cook for 15 minutes, stirring occasionally.

When the curry is ready, remove from the heat and add in coconut yoghurt for extra creaminess if you prefer.

Garnish with fresh coriander and serve with fluffy basmati rice and vegan parathas.

MEATLESS TIKKA MASALA

SERVES 4

1 x 400g tin young, green jackfruit in water/brine
1 x 400g tin chopped tomatoes
1 x 400g tin coconut milk
1 medium onion, chopped
6-8 garlic cloves, finely chopped
1 teaspoon cumin seeds
1 teaspoon chilli powder
1 teaspoon ground coriander
1 teaspoon garam masala
½ teaspoon cinnamon
vegetable oil
fresh coriander to garnish
coconut yoghurt (optional)

Healthy Indian food at home that's better than a takeaway. It's creamy, spicy, and meaty despite being completely plant-based! Enjoy with fluffy basmati rice and vegan parathas.

Preheat the oven to 200°C (400°F).

Rinse and drain the jackfruit, then cut into smaller, bite-sizes.

Mix the chilli powder, coriander, cinnamon and garam masala in a large bowl. Tip in the jackfruit pieces in and coat on all sides.

Spread the seasoned jackfruit out on a lightly greased baking sheet and bake for 20 minutes.

Meanwhile, pour 1 tablespoon of vegetable oil in a large saucepan on a medium heat. Add the cumin seeds for 1-2 minutes until they begin to crack. Add the chopped onion and garlic and cook for 3-5 minutes until soft.

Add the jackfruit from the oven into the pan and stir for 1-2 minutes. Next, add in the chopped tomatoes and coconut milk. Mix well, then cover and reduce the heat to simmer. Leave to cook for 15 minutes, stirring occasionally.

When the curry is ready, remove from the heat and add in coconut yoghurt for extra creaminess if you prefer.

Garnish with fresh coriander and serve with fluffy basmati rice and vegan parathas.

SMOKY PULLED-NOT-PORK TACOS

SERVES 4
FOR THE FILLING
2 x 400g tins young, green jackfruit in water/brine
2 tablespoons coconut oil
½ onion, thinly sliced
4 garlic cloves, minced
1 tablespoon smoked paprika
1 tablespoon ground cumin
1 tablespoon chilli powder
2-3 tablespoons maple syrup
1-2 red or green chillies, chopped
3 teaspoons hot habanero sauce
3 tablespoons lime juice
FOR SERVING
8 tacos
1 x 400g tin refried pinto or black beans
chopped avocado
fresh coriander
lime wedges
salsa
hot habanero sauce

Tacos have become one of the most popular recipes to make with jackfruit, and there's a reason for it – they're so tasty! The meatiness of the jackfruit perfectly marries with the crunchiness of the tacos. Go wild with the heat you handle. Any leftover jackfruit can be stored in the fridge for 4-5 days or frozen and defrosted overnight before cooking.

Rinse and drain the jackfruit. Transfer to a chopping board and cut into small pieces. Pull the pieces apart with either a fork or your fingers to resemble pulled pork.

Heat a large frying pan over medium heat with a tablespoon of coconut oil. Once hot, add in the chopped onion, garlic, and chillies. Cook for 4-5 minutes until fragrant and the onions have softened.

Add the jackfruit to the pan along with the paprika, cumin, chilli powder, maple syrup and lime juice. Coat the jackfruit in the spices and cook for 3-5 minutes. Add in 50ml of water then reduce the heat and cover for 20 minutes, stirring occasionally.

As your jackfruit is cooking and begins to soften, you can continue to break up the pieces with a fork or a spoon to give it more of a 'stringy' pulled meat effect.

Taste and adjust the flavour as needed – add some habanero sauce for spiciness, more paprika for smokiness, or lime juice for acidity. Cook for a further 2-3 minutes then remove from heat. Serve up in tacos with toppings of your choice – I love refried beans, salsa and extra habanero sauce!

STICKY JACKFRUIT RIBS

SERVES 4

1 x 400g tin young, green jackfruit in water/brine
80ml vegan BBQ sauce plus extra for serving
150g wheat gluten flour (seitan)
2 tablespoons tamari
3 tablespoons tahini
3 tablespoons nutritional yeast
1 tablespoon smoked paprika
1 garlic clove, minced
salt and pepper

I've tried to push jackfruit to the limit with the recipes in this book and these 'ribs' are something I was really proud of. Serve them wrapped in foil over a summer BBQ for extra deliciousness. They can also be made in advance and frozen, just defrost overnight before cooking.

Heat a non-stick pan over medium-high heat. Drain and rinse the jackfruit then add to the pan. Cook for 1-2 minutes then add the BBQ sauce and 3-4 tablespoons of water. Lower the heat, cover and simmer for 10-12 minutes. Give it a stir every few minutes and start to break up the jackfruit with a fork as it softens so the fibres absorb more of the sauce.

Remove the cover and continue to mash the jackfruit with a fork or a potato masher. If any tough pieces of jackfruit remain, simply put them on a cutting board and thinly slice. Leave the jackfruit to cool completely.

Preheat the oven to 190°C (350°F).

Meanwhile, combine the wheat gluten flour, nutritional yeast, smoked paprika, and a pinch of salt and pepper in a large bowl and combine. Then add 150ml water, tamari, cooled jackfruit, and tahini. Mix well and then knead until all ingredients are evenly distributed and absorbed. If it feels too dry, add one or two tablespoons of water.

Oil a medium baking dish. Spread the jackfruit mixture evenly across the bottom and cut into desired number of ribs (it should make around 16 ribs). Bake for 30 minutes.

Remove from the oven and use a knife to loosen along the edges along the tray. Brush the top of the mixture with BBQ sauce and then flip over in the dish. Coat the other side (now the top) with BBQ sauce and return to the oven. Bake for another 25-30 minutes. The 'ribs' should be firm and cooked in the middle. Brush with more BBQ sauce if desired and serve immediately.

TERIYAKI BOWL

SERVES 4
FOR THE TERIYAKI JACKFRUIT
1 x 400g tin young, green jackfruit in brine
1 garlic clove, minced
1 thumb-sized piece of ginger, peeled and chopped
1 teaspoon sesame oil
3 tablespoons brown sugar
4 tablespoons tamari
6 tablespoons rice vinegar
2 tablespoons toasted sesame seeds
ACCOMPANIMENTS
500g spinach, wilted
1 large carrot, peeled into ribbons
170g basmati rice
2-3 teaspoons pickled ginger (optional)
1 avocado, sliced (optional)
60g watercress (optional)

Fix your cravings for Asian takeaway with this perfectly balanced teriyaki jackfruit rice bowl. Canned jackfruit in brine works slightly better for this recipe as the saltiness compliments the teriyaki sweetness.

Place a pan of water on to boil. Cook the rice for 10 minutes. Drain and set aside to cool.

Drain and rinse the jackfruit. Place the jackfruit chunks in a non-stick frying pan over a medium-high heat. Allow all sides to slightly golden but be careful not to break the jackfruit up too much as you want it to stay in chunks as much as possible.

Combine the garlic, ginger, sesame oil, brown sugar, tamari, and rice vinegar in a small bowl. Add to the jackfruit and leave to simmer over a medium heat for around 8 minutes until it reduces to a thicker glaze.

Prepare the carrots. Cut the carrot in half lengthwise. Then, using a vegetable peeler, shave thin but wide slices. Wrap them around each other to form a simple rose. Secure using a toothpick.

Heat a dry frying pan over a medium heat and add the spinach until it wilts.

Assemble the rice, spinach, jackfruit and carrot roses in a bowl. Sprinkle with sesame seeds and serve with additional toppings of pickled ginger, avocado, or watercress.

FISH-FREE FINGERS AND CHIPS

SERVES 4
FOR THE FISH-FREE FINGERS
1 x 400g tin young, green jackfruit in water/brine
1 x 400g tin chickpeas
2 x sushi nori sheets
1 leek, finely sliced
1 teaspoon vegetable oil
salt and pepper
50g breadcrumbs
1 lemon cut into wedges, to serve
FOR THE TARTAR SAUCE
175g veganaise
1 shallot, finely diced
1 tablespoon capers, drained
1 tablespoon gherkins, finely chopped
1 tablespoon lemon juice
½ tablespoon chopped parsley
½ tablespoon chopped dill
salt and pepper

The secret to this 'fishiness' is using nori seaweed strips. Serve with homemade vegan tartar sauce and salad or hand cut potato chips.

Make the tartar sauce first by combining all the ingredients and mixing them well. Sprinkle extra dill on top for decoration. Refrigerate until you are ready to use it.

Toast the nori sheets in a dry frying pan on a high heat for 1-2 minutes until they start to go black and crumble. Set aside.

Drain and rinse the jackfruit. Add the jackfruit and nori to a food processor and mix until the jackfruit starts to flake but not for too long that it becomes mushy. Put the mixture in a large bowl.

Heat a teaspoon of vegetable oil on a low heat and fry the sliced leeks for 3-5 minutes until soft. Transfer to the food processor along with the chickpeas, a pinch of salt and pepper, and blend until smooth. Add to the large bowl with the jackfruit and mix everything well.

Pour the breadcrumbs on to a plate. Take one tablespoon of the jackfruit mixture, squeeze between your hands (this will hold them together more when cooking) into an oblong finger shape, and then roll in the breadcrumbs. Do this with all of the mixture.

Pour a thin layer of vegetable oil in a wide frying pan and heat until very hot. Fry the 'fish' fingers on each side till browned and crispy. Drain on kitchen roll to get rid of any excess oil. Serve with the tartar sauce, a lemon wedge, and a side salad or hand-cut potato chips.

THAI FISH-FREE CAKES

MAKES 6 'FISH' CAKES
FOR THE 'FISH CAKES'
1 x 400g tin young, green jackfruit in water/brine
2 medium potatoes
1 tablespoon sesame oil
2 tablespoons red Thai curry paste
3 spring onions, thinly sliced
1 thumb-sized piece of ginger, peeled and chopped
1 tablespoon tamari
1 tablespoon fresh coriander, chopped
100g panko breadcrumbs
FOR THE SAUCE
1 tablespoon toasted sesame seeds
2 tablespoons tamari
2 tablespoons lime juice
1 tablespoon fresh coriander, chopped
1 teaspoon sugar
½ red chilli, finely chopped

Hot, spicy and wonderfully moreish. Whilst potato isn't a traditional Thai ingredient, it's what my Mum always used for fish cakes and it works as a perfect binder for the jackfruit Serve with our dipping sauce and a side salad for a deliciously light dinner.

First, make the dipping sauce by mixing together all the ingredients in a small dish. Set aside.
Bring a large pan of water to boil. Peel the potatoes, cut them into large cubes and boil for 15 minutes. Drain and mash well.
Heat a tablespoon of sesame oil in a frying pan on a medium heat. Add the sliced spring onions and chopped ginger. Cook for 2-3 minutes until fragrant.
Drain and rinse the jackfruit, roughly chop and add to the frying pan with the onions and ginger. Fry for 5 minutes, stirring so the pieces are covered.
Add the red Thai curry paste, reduce the heat to low medium and fry for a further 15 minutes, stirring regularly. Use a fork to break the jackfruit pieces up so that the fibres absorb more of the paste. Add the mashed potato and mix together well. Remove the pan from the heat.
Tip the panko breadcrumbs on to a plate. Using a spoon (or your your hands if the mixture has cooled down), form the mixture into 6 patties. Coat the outside of each with panko breadcrumbs. Heat a tablespoon of oil in a non-stick pan on a medium heat. Let the oil get really hot, then add the patties to the pan and fry for a few minutes on each side until golden brown. srve the 'fish' cakes with the dipping sauce and a sprinkling of coriander